STRENGTH TRAINING FOR COACHES

Bruno Pauletto, MS
University of Tennessee

Leisure Press
Champaign, Illinois

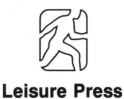

Library of Congress Cataloging-in-Publication Data

Pauletto, Bruno, 1954-
    Strength training for coaches / by Bruno Pauletto.
      p.   cm.
    Includes bibliographical references (p.).
    ISBN 0-88011-371-5
    1. Weight training. 2. Coaches (Athletics)   I. Title.
    GV546.P295   1991
    613.7'13--dc20   90-13122
                                    CIP

ISBN: 0-88011-371-5

Acquisitions Editor: Brian Holding
Developmental Editors: June I. Decker, PhD, and Robert King
Assistant Editors: Julia Anderson, Dawn Levy, and Kari Nelson
Copyeditor: Barbara Walsh
Proofreaders: Pam Johnson and David Severtson
Production Director: Ernie Noa
Typesetter: Yvonne Winsor
Text Design: Keith Blomberg
Text Layout: Tara Welsch
Cover Design: Hunter Graphics
Cover Photo: Wilmer Zehr
Interior Photos: Nick Myers
Models: David Hawkins, William Hudson, and Lisa Stegman
Printer: Versa Press

Leisure Press books are available at special discounts for bulk purchase for sales promotions, premiums, fund-raising, or educational use. Special editions or book excerpts can also be created to specification. For details, contact the Special Sales Manager at Leisure Press.

Printed in the United States of America

10 9 8 7 6 5 4 3 2

Leisure Press
A Division of Human Kinetics Publishers, Inc.
Box 5076, Champaign, IL 61825-5076
1-800-747-4457

Canada Office:
Human Kinetics Publishers, Inc.
P.O. Box 2503, Windsor, ON N8Y 4S2
1-800-465-7301 (in Canada only)

Europe Office:
Human Kinetics Publishers (Europe) Ltd.
P.O. Box IW14
Leeds LS16 6TR
England 0532-781708

Australia Office:
Human Kinetics Publishers
P.O. Box 80
Kingswood 5062
South Australia 374-0433

To Jesus Christ, my personal savior.

Contents

Preface

In recent years strength training has become an integral part of most sport programs. We now recognize that improving muscular strength through a good strength program not only helps our athletes perform better in their sports but helps reduce the number and seriousness of injuries. It is no longer a question of *whether* to strength train but rather *how* it can be done best.

Strength training is much more than just "pumping iron." It is a well-planned, systematic process designed to improve total body strength. It is used to make your linemen become stronger, your high jumper jump higher, your sprinter run faster, or your wrestler keep 'em pinned to the mat. In fact, strength training is used every day in every sport to make athletes the best they can be. As coaches, we need to ask ourselves whether we are using strength training to the best advantage.

Whether you coach intermediate, high school, or college athletes, this book is written for you, the coach. I have tried to address all aspects of strength training, from setting up your facilities and creating a program that will work best within your facility, to teaching the exercises. Because of its broad coverage and detailed information, this book is beneficial to *all sports at any level*.

Chapter 1, "Your Facility," gives information to improve your existing facility and what

to consider when building a facility from scratch.

Chapter 2, "Equipment," contains suggestions for how to upgrade your equipment and keep it in good working order, what to look for in new equipment, the pros and cons of free weights and machines, and even how to make your own equipment.

Chapter 3, "Organizing Your Program," suggests how to balance the number of athletes you have with the amount of time, space, and equipment available. You will find suggestions about coaching a large number of athletes with limited human resources.

Chapter 4, "Weight Room Safety," covers weight room rules and procedures, spotting techniques, and the facility itself. Out of concern for our athletes and because of the liability consciousness in the world today, you must keep your weight room and strength training program safe. Rules and regulations must be made and enforced.

Chapter 5, "Motivation," deals with various methods of motivation—intrinsic (that from within the athlete) and extrinsic (motivation that can be applied outwardly)—that can help lead your athletes to optimal strength workouts.

Chapter 6, "Strength Training Principles," simplifies, for your understanding, the general principles of strength training that have been proven to work. This chapter includes information about muscles, rest, overtraining, and how hard and how often to train your athletes.

Chapter 7, "Classic Circuit Training," explains how this type of training can be applied to suit your needs. Circuit strength training is very popular because it allows a coach to train a large number of athletes with very little time and equipment.

Chapter 8, "Designing Your Own Program," takes you step by step through the design of your own strength training program. Considerations are given to different sports, time available, and limitations you may encounter.

Chapter 9, "Testing and Evaluation," offers advice on how to test, when to test, and what to do with the test results.

Chapters 10, 11, and 12, on the core exercises, cover the proper technique of the basic core exercises used to develop total-body strength and describe the benefits of each exercise. Each exercise technique is explained in full, and a complete photo sequence showing the correct technique and the most common errors accompanies the text. A checklist follows each core exercise to aid you as you train your athletes.

Chapter 13, "Auxiliary Exercises," covers a large variety of auxiliary exercises organized by muscle group. The exercises are explained and described in detail and are accompanied by photos demonstrating how the exercises are done.

The Glossary at the end of the book defines terms that you may not be familiar with.

Acknowledgments

Thanks to my wife, Julie, for the support, dedication, and hard work that helped make this book possible.

A special thanks to

- the staff at Human Kinetics;
- my many coaching friends throughout the country who through the years have helped broaden my experience in the field;
- Nick Myers for the great job he did with the photographs;
- Models David Hawkins, William Hudson, and Lisa Stegman; and
- Phil Emery for his help in the final review.

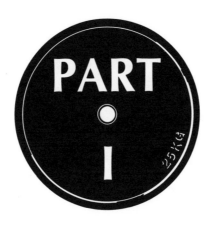

PROGRAM ADMINISTRATION

Your Facility

We all know that to accomplish a task one needs the right tools. The better job you do in developing your strength facility and equipment, the better chance you have in building a successful strength program. A modern and continually upgraded facility helps everyone who uses it. Facility improvements involve both the physical space and the equipment in it. This chapter deals with your space and chapter 2 with the specifics of equipment.

UPGRADING AN EXISTING FACILITY

Improving an existing facility is a never-ending project. Every year there are things to do—painting, cleaning the carpets, even moving a wall and expanding. Like many of us, you may have limited space and little money to do anything about it. In this chapter I'll give you ideas for spending your money wisely.

Whatever dollars you have each year, from gate receipts, fund-raising, or budget allocations, need to be spent carefully. If you can make only a few improvements each year, have a long-range plan to reach your ultimate goal. This means you will not have everything you need right away, but by careful planning you should get there in a few years.

Here are some suggestions to help you with your long-range planning.

It takes equipment to get your athletes strong, so that should be your first priority. Even if your room is not very pretty you will get great results with the right equipment.

Do not replace old equipment if it can be refurbished. Only after you have everything you need should old equipment be replaced with better. For example, you may have an old plate-loaded lat pull-down machine, in good shape but not very practical. Keep it and spend your money buying additional pieces of equipment that are needed more urgently. When you can, replace it with a new, modern selectorized model. (See chapter 2 on ''Equipment'' for more tips.)

After your basic needs in equipment are met, spend some of your money on beautifying your room. You may want to paint the walls, replace the carpet, buy more mats, or improve the lighting. Do what is most important first and then next year do more. (The next section, on customizing the weight room, gives more guidance in this area.)

Say that for several years you have been improving the weight room little by little. Your room looks good; you have the basic equipment you need but have no further floor space to continue expanding. The ultimate solution would be to have a new, larger weight room built, but for most coaches this is improbable. If you *can* build a new facility, refer to the next section of this chapter. If not, you might expand by tearing down walls and incorporating an adjacent room. Or you might move the weight room to a larger space in another part of the building. Good planning and support from school administration can make either of these possible. If you are considering expansion, study the points I discuss for building a new weight room, because many could apply to expanding existing space.

BUILDING A NEW FACILITY

In most cases it will be a frosty day in July before you get a brand-new weight room. I have noticed, though, that more and more schools are putting in new weight rooms. This section deals with building a new facility when funds are available and the project has been approved. If you are getting a new facility, good for you! You should find this section helpful.

Building a new weight room is exciting. You can't wait to work in a new facility. You can just imagine more space, new equipment, clean floors, a new stereo, and all the things you've dreamed about for years. But for this to become reality you have to take an active part in building the new weight room. If you sit back and expect these things to just happen, you will be deeply disappointed. Get excited and get involved!

The Making of a Weight Room

When a new weight room is first mentioned, it is time for action. There is a lot to be done before the first construction worker sets foot on the property. You need to give your expertise to the people in charge so the weight room is done correctly and suits your needs. I have found that the people in charge (architects, school officials, etc.) usually do not really understand the practicalities of a weight room. They know the construction of buildings but do not fully comprehend what actually goes on in a weight room and how the physical components of the room can help the athletes. The following guidelines will assist you at each step of the way.

Research

When you are asked to give your input as to size, layout, and location, you need to have as much information ready as possible. Start by looking at what other people have done, and learn from this information. Visit several facilities, high school or college, and take notes on what you like or do not like. Talk with the coaches about the problems they encountered during the building of their weight rooms or what they might have done differently. Compile all this information to give yourself a clearer idea of what you can do and what to expect. Develop your own checklist of what is important and how to get it done.

Assessing Needs

Using all the information you have compiled, assess your own needs. Make sure the room will fulfill your present and future needs. Keep these points in mind.

Location. Is the room separate or within the structure of the school building? Is it easily accessible to the athletes? Are the other facilities nearby (e.g., gym, office, bathrooms, playing field)? The closer the weight room is to these facilities, the better.

Number of Users. Determine the number of students who will use the weight room. Take into consideration all varsity sports, physical education classes, and student activities. The weight room must accommodate the needs of the whole school.

Equipment. What kind of equipment will be used, and what is the total number of pieces you will have? The more training stations you expect to include, the more room you will need. Free-weight equipment generally takes up more room than machines because of space needed for plate storage, loading and unloading the bars, and spotting.

Costs. Before you submit your ideas, try to find out how much money is available for the facility. Estimate how much you think your ideas will cost. Find out if what you have in mind fits into the general scheme of things. You may have to scale down your expectations if there is not enough money available.

If you do not know how much is available, supply estimates for what you think should be done. The estimate should include all of what you would like plus a cushion of about 10% for unpredictable expenses. Remember that building a new facility is a one-time shot, and you want it to be the best and most efficient facility possible.

Proposal Presentation

Once you know quite well what you need, present a proposal to the people in charge. It should be very detailed in all its calculations and should take into consideration every aspect of the new building or area. (See page 6 in this chapter, "Customizing the Weight Room.") If possible give some options in case compromises are necessary. State the reasons you want certain things, and use examples of and comparisons to what you have seen at other schools. Do not assume people understand the reasons for your requests.

This first proposal should be only for the structure (Figure 1.1). You may need an additional proposal for the equipment and furnishings (Figure 1.2).

Compromise

Your proposal may not be accepted as is because of costs or because the architect decides it does not fit into the plans. You will probably be asked to work with the architect to design a room that fits into the plan and falls within the budget allocated for the project. At this time,

---

(*Date*)

(*Name of person proposal is directed to*)

Proposal issued from:

(*Your name and title*)

(*Your school name*)

Based on the number of students who presently use our weight room facility, we need to expand to 1,500 square feet. This can be achieved by expanding into and taking over an adjacent room. Several schools in our district have facilities similar to or larger than the one I propose. They are the following:

1. Central High School
2. St. Mary's High School
3. Hancock High School

The following information will help you see just how much we need the extra room:

Number of students who will use the facility	500
Number of varsity sports using the facility	12
Number of strength physical education classes	4 per day
Average number of students in facility at any given time	35
Total hours room is used daily	9
Square footage of present facility	1,000

The new facility should have the following features:

1. Carpeted floor (Give specifics: e.g., Mr. Porter, father of Kevin Porter, will install the carpet for free.)
2. Rubberized dumbbell area (Give size and cost along with reasons why you need the area.)

(*List any other physical parts of the weight room you want improved and their approximate costs.*)

Total estimated cost for expansion and upgrading:

$ _____

Figure 1.1 Sample proposal for facility enhancement.

List all old equipment you intend to keep.
Give estimated cost to refurbish the old
    equipment.
List all new equipment needed.
Give estimated cost to purchase new
    equipment.
Give reasons for your decision.

Figure 1.2   Items to include in an equipment proposal.

the knowledge you have accumulated during your research becomes critical. Dozens of decisions about things like floor covering, lights, and air conditioning will be made. The more you know and the more information you can give, the better.

Weight Room Layout

After the size and location of your weight room have been determined, you need to plan the room layout. Seeing what other people have done and knowing what will suit your needs gives you a good idea of what to do.

Leave enough space around the equipment for the athletes to move around without disturbing each other. An athlete should be able to train on a piece of equipment without interfering with the adjacent trainee. Each piece of equipment will use approximately 50 square feet of your room. If your room is approximately 1,000 square feet you will be able to have about 20 pieces of equipment. Free-weight equipment (e.g., squat) will usually take up more room than machines (e.g., leg press). You will need specific aisles and open areas. Room should also be left for spotting and changing plates. For example, do not place a bar too close to a wall; leave at least 2 feet between the bar and the wall for changing plates.

Do not put equipment in the way of traffic areas, such as near water fountains, entrance doors, office doors, and strength training areas.

The sequence of equipment placement should save steps. The athlete should not have to travel back and forth unnecessarily to complete a workout. Place the equipment to suit your needs. The following considerations will help (see sample floor plans in Figure 1.3, a–c):

- If you will be using circuit training, arrange the equipment in the order in which you want the athletes to do the exercises, so athletes can move easily and quickly from one station to another.
- If you emphasize a split routine (different body parts are trained on different days), put all the equipment pertaining to upper body parts in one vicinity and equipment for lower body parts in another. This allows the athlete to stay in one particular area of the weight room and do a full workout while in the other part of the room another group is training different body parts.
- You can designate a specific area for core exercises and another smaller area for all the auxiliary exercises. Usually, you have several pieces of core exercise apparatus (e.g., bench press) but only one or two pieces of auxiliary exercise apparatus (e.g., neck machines).
- Keep in mind how you will supervise the weight room. If a few exercises are of major concern to you, you might want to keep that exercise equipment in one area so that you can better supervise those exercises.

To determine where the equipment should be and whether it will fit in the desired area, draw a floor plan (to scale) on graph paper. Then draw equipment to scale on cardboard and cut out the pieces. Each piece represents the size and shape of the equipment. Place the pieces on your floor plan and make any changes you want by moving pieces around to see where they fit best. When you have reached a final decision, glue the pieces in place. This will serve as a diagram when you are ready to set up the room. Some large equipment companies can do a computerized floor plan for you (Figure 1.3).

CUSTOMIZING THE WEIGHT ROOM

I have compiled a basic checklist of items you might want to consider when building or remodeling your facility.

Room Shape

The room should be square or rectangular with no pillars or other blind spots. If you cannot avoid having blind spots, make them useful by attaching equipment or mirrors to them. You should be able to see the entire room from any

Space required: 875 square ft

Scale 1/8″ = 1′0″

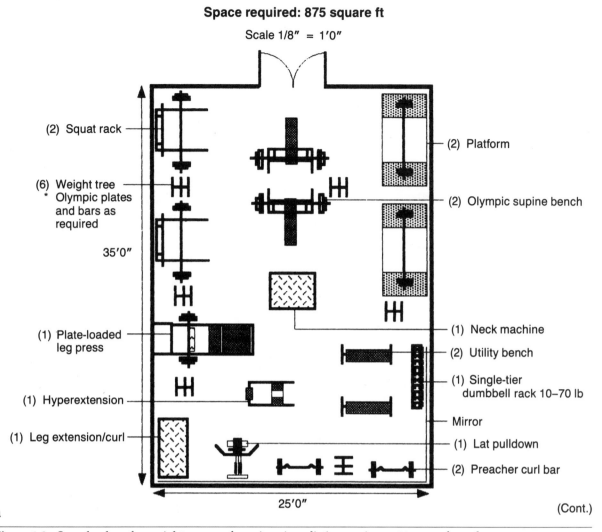

a

(Cont.)

Figure 1.3 Sample plans for weight rooms of varying sizes, listing equipment type and number.

point within it. Try to have one large, open area, not a series of small rooms. Eliminate all unnecessary obstructions.

Ceiling

The ceiling should be high enough to clear the equipment (suggested minimum: 11 feet). A higher ceiling gives the room a more open feeling. If you have an unfinished, open ceiling, try to add an inexpensive drop ceiling to reduce room noise and enhance the room's appearance.

Floor

The floor should be made of reinforced concrete to support the heavy load of equipment. Be cautious if floor supports are made of wood or if the weight room is not on the ground floor. Ideally, the entire floor should be rubberized. Rub-

ber keeps feet from slipping and protects the floor if weights are dropped. If rubberizing the entire floor is too costly, do it in the areas where weights are likely to be dropped (e.g., during pulling exercises, dumbbells). One inexpensive way to buy rubber is to purchase an old rubber conveyor belt from a heavy industrial company. Carpet is second-best; if you use carpet, choose a short-pile industrial grade. It is easier to clean than a higher pile and safer because it does not grab the soles of shoes. Tiles and bare concrete are poor choices because they can be slippery when wet, creating a hazard.

Walls

Walls made of regular concrete block make it easy to install wall-mounted equipment. Paint them with a washable paint in a light color to make the room look larger and brighter. Use

Space required: 1,200 square ft

Scale 1/8″ = 1′0″

(1) Neck machine

(1) Hyperextension

(3) Squat rack

(3) Platform

(4) Olympic supine bench

(9) Weight tree
* Olympic plates and bars as required

40′0″

(1) Plate-loaded leg press

(1) Leg curl

(1) Leg extension

(1) Wall-mount chin-up

(1) Double-dip stand

Mirror

Utility bench

(1) Preacher curl bench

(1) Two-tier dumbbell rack 10–80 lb

b

(1) Lat pulldowr

30′0″

(3) Preacher curl bar

(Cont.)

Figure 1.3   (Continued)

the walls to your advantage by affixing equipment, mirrors, bulletin boards, motivational material, and painted-on logos.

Windows

Windows let in natural light and fresh air, but you must make sure the room is arranged so that there is no direct sunlight on the athletes. Trainees will be disturbed by the sun shining in their faces while they perform exercises. If your room gets direct sunlight, install tinted glass windows or cover the windows with blinds.

Doors

Double doors into the weight room make it easier to move equipment in and out and make the room look bigger. If there is a center post in the double doors, it should be removable.

Ventilation

The best temperature for a weight room is about 68 degrees. Central heating/air conditioning is the best choice; there should be as many air vents as possible to distribute air evenly. If no

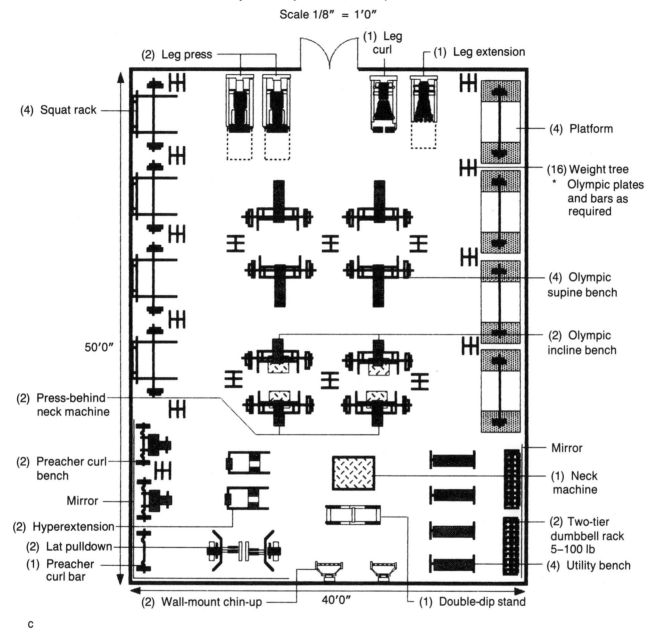

Space Required: 2,000 square ft

Scale 1/8″ = 1′0″

(1) Leg curl
(1) Leg extension
(2) Leg press
(4) Squat rack
(4) Platform
(16) Weight tree
  * Olympic plates and bars as required
(4) Olympic supine bench
(2) Olympic incline bench
50′0″
(2) Press-behind neck machine
Mirror
(2) Preacher curl bench
(1) Neck machine
Mirror
(2) Two-tier dumbbell rack 5–100 lb
(2) Hyperextension
(2) Lat pulldown
(1) Preacher curl bar
(4) Utility bench
(2) Wall-mount chin-up
40′0″
(1) Double-dip stand

c

Figure 1.3 (Continued)

central system is available use a number of fans to circulate the air. On mild days open the windows or let in fresh air any way you can.

Music

Music is a great motivator for young athletes. If you can, install a good central system with an AM/FM radio, a cassette player, and several speakers spread evenly around the room. Secure the system in an office or storage area. If a central system is out of the question, use a regular portable unit (boom box). Avoid using just a few large speakers because an athlete who is too close to them cannot hear what is going on. This is a safety hazard.

Mirrors

Mirrors make a room brighter and appear larger. Use as many as you can but not in areas where they might disrupt the lifters. If you place mirrors near squats or platforms, athletes tend to watch themselves do the exercises instead of feeling the movements. But for certain exercises like arm curls, mirrors can help athletes as they watch their arms get pumped up. Mirrors should be 1 or 2 feet off the floor and stand 7 to 8 feet tall. For continuity place them side by side and try to cover the whole wall or area. Choose glass mirrors over plastic ones, which tend to be distorted and unclear.

Office

If you are in charge of the weight room full time your office should be in the weight room near the main entrance. It should have a large window facing the weight room so that you can observe the room when you are working at your desk. If your office is elsewhere in the building you may want to have a small work area in the weight room (e.g., a desk in the corner) as well as a storage closet for your materials.

Storage

It is important to have a storage room in or near the weight room. It should be large enough to store extra equipment so it is not left lying around the weight room. If it is large enough you can also use it as a place to repair equipment.

Electrical Outlets

Have several outlets (110 volt) spread around the room. You may need them for music, video equipment, fans, or special lighting for filming. Equipment installed in the future may need 220-volt electrical power, so include a few of these outlets as well.

Lighting

The lighting should be bright enough to make the room inviting and safe. Good lighting also enables you to use video equipment and shoot pictures at any time. If possible, install full-spectrum lighting. Control switches should be near the entrance or in the office.

Water Fountain

Water should always be readily available to the trainees. The fountain should be located in or very close to the weight room so you can keep tight control of the athletes. They will make several trips to the water fountain during workouts.

Rest Rooms

Rest rooms should also be located in or very close to the weight room. Such placement will discourage athletes from using rest room excuses to delay exercises and prolong workouts.

Entrance Area

This area will have your bulletin board, workout pickup boxes, belt pickup, and weight scale. All this should be located so as not to interfere with in-and-out traffic. Also near the entrance area should be an area for stretching. If space is not available right in the weight room, it should be very close by.

Decoration

Make your room attractive. Use pictures, posters, wall graphics, and so on. A positive atmosphere creates a positive attitude, which promotes further strength gains.

FUND-RAISING

A portion of your school system's regular physical education or athletic budget should be set aside for weight room improvement and acquisition of new equipment. Also, a portion of the booster club donations should be used for maintenance of the weight room. These funds are not always available and even if they are, they usually do not provide enough money to meet the needs of an expanding strength and conditioning program. In these days of budget cuts and reallocation, most programs must rely on fund-raising to expand or improve their weight rooms. It is up to the coach, athletes, and other interested individuals to bring in extra revenue for desired projects. Whatever you do, be sure you give credit to whoever has helped. Make sure you have insurance for these events. Here are a few suggestions for fund-raising.

Lift-a-Thon

Athletes get pledges for the number of pounds they lift in the lift-a-thon. They are given a specific length of time to solicit pledges from individuals, businesses, and organizations. All pledges must be collected after the lift-a-thon in a specific time period. If your group collects 90% of its pledges, you are doing very well. The most popular exercise used in a lift-a-thon is the bench press.

Divide the athletes into teams; form some kind of competition and reward the winners (e.g., the team that raised the most money).

Clubs

Organize a lifting club at your school. Students can come and lift for physical well-being or physical appearance. Charge the students a small fee to use the facilities. Make the room available when workouts or classes are not in session. You or another qualified individual will supervise the club.

Sell a Product

Athletes can sell T-shirts, candy bars, calendars, or other items. Use the revenues to improve the weight room.

Competition

You may want to organize a lifting competition in the school. All participants pay a fee; you can also charge spectators a small fee. After meeting the expenses for prizes and awards, you should still have a net income when the competition is over.

Car Wash

Hold a car wash at a local service station. The cost of soap, buckets, and sponges is minimal.

Parent Skills

This is not a money-gathering drive but a rally of ''human power.'' Have your athletes hold a drive to get parents to donate their time and expertise to improving the weight room. This would make materials your only cost. In some cases even the materials may be donated. For example, a local carpet merchant may install the carpet for free, or the father of one of the athletes who is a painter can paint the room. The services are limited only by the ability of you and your athletes to generate interest in your program.

CHAPTER 2

Equipment

Now that you have a better understanding of the physical components of a weight room, let's look at the most important part of that room: the equipment. You need a weight room with a variety of equipment for strength training the total body. Rarely will a coach be able to get all the needed equipment in a single purchase. In most cases a few pieces are bought each year. Therefore, buy the equipment you need the most so your dollars are well spent. The sample floor plans in chapter 1 show some basic equipment needs. Of course, you will buy according to your facility size and budget limitations.

BUYING EQUIPMENT

Certified strength and conditioning coaches are well qualified to advise you regarding your needs. You can find your nearest certified strength and conditioning specialist by contacting the National Strength and Conditioning Association (P.O. Box 81410, Lincoln, NE, 68501, 402-472-3000). Do not be afraid to consult with these specialists; they are usually happy to help. Unless you already know exactly what you want, you have much to gain from their experience.

Afterward, consult with different dealers to see what they have to offer. Ask them a series of questions as shown in Figure 2.1. Naturally,

each dealer will recommend his or her own product as the best on the market or the most complete. An even better source may be a dealer who represents several manufacturers. This person may be more likely to find equipment to fit your specifications and budget.

1. Do you have the specific equipment I need?
2. Do you have different models of the particular piece of equipment?
3. How much does it cost?
4. How much are the shipping costs?
5. Can it be painted in my school colors, and if so, at what extra cost?
6. What is the time of delivery after the order is sent in?
7. What kind of warranty applies?
8. Who unloads the equipment off the delivery truck?
9. Can you give me some references of people you have sold equipment to?
10. Why is your product the best for the money?

Figure 2.1 Ten questions to ask equipment dealers.

Equipment Dealers

I have often found that when the time comes to buy equipment, many coaches do not know where to turn. The local equipment dealer is not always the best option.

Start creating a file of different dealers, companies you can turn to when you need equipment. You should have a variety of options so you can get the best possible equipment for the money you have to spend. Here are several sources of information.

- When dealers come to visit your school, keep their information and business cards.
- Clinics, conventions, and exhibitions always have several booths representing different equipment manufacturers. Attend some of these and gather information.
- Keep brochures and catalogs that come through the mail. You may not need equipment now, but when you do you will have this information at hand to facilitate your decision.

Buying Hints

Most public schools have state regulations that require the coach to present a requisition to the school board (see Figure 2.2). The requisition is sent to different companies for bids. The company that can furnish the equipment at the lowest price is awarded the order. In most states, when the total is less than a specific amount (e.g., $300) the coach can purchase the equipment outright without going through the bidding process. Check with your school board to see how to proceed.

Schools not regulated by the state (i.e., private schools) may be able to purchase any amount of equipment outright if approved by the athletic director or other authority.

Whether or not you are submitting the purchase for bids, be very precise when you present a requisition or an order for equipment. For example, if you want a bench press, state all the particulars (size, color, style, construction material, quality of padding, unit price: see the section on equipment specifications on page 16). If you are not specific, the salesperson may submit bids for or send equipment that is very different or considerably lower in quality than what you expect.

If possible, buy locally or in your region. You will save money on freight, especially if you buy several pieces of equipment. You can also have a closer relationship with the manufacturer, making maintenance or repairs easier to obtain.

A smaller company may be more service-oriented than a larger company. Small does not always mean unknown or beginning. Small companies are usually still growing and eager to have their product in the marketplace, so they may give better deals. Do be sure they are dependable and have the necessary credibility and product liability insurance. Large, well-known companies stand behind their products and often have regional dealers you can contact.

The price quoted to you should include delivery and installation. But if you want to save money, you might be interested in picking up and installing the equipment yourself. You must always be sure the price you are quoted is clear as to what it covers.

Be wary of complete weight room deals a company offers at substantial savings. One company may not carry the best products in all lines. It may have good machines but poor bars and weights. Break down the total purchase into smaller parts (e.g., machines, free weights, bars, plates, dumbbells, floor mats). If you buy from a variety of equipment companies you will more likely get quality merchandise in all areas. More often than not, super deals mean inferior quality.

Get complete information on equipment guarantees or warrantees (see "Ten Questions to Ask Equipment Dealers," Figure 2.1 in this chapter). Get an exact delivery date. Can your equipment be delivered on time? Ask around to see if the company is dependable or if it has a reputation for failing to meet delivery deadlines.

If the equipment is to be shipped, how will it be shipped? Who is responsible if equipment is damaged when it arrives? Damaged goods are usually the delivery company's responsibility, but you often have to go through lengthy procedures to correct the situation. By law, you have a number of days, usually 60 to 90, to make a claim against the shipper or originator. In the meantime, you are stuck with defective equipment you cannot use.

All equipment is fragile, even weight training equipment. Paint can be scratched, upholstery torn, rods and frames bent. Check all equipment before you sign it off as delivered. Look for scratches, tears, or bends, and make sure that pulleys and moving parts operate smoothly. Be sure you have exactly the equipment you requested in the purchase order, and

School Name

Requisition   Requisition number _____

                                         Date _____

Vendor: _____   Need delivery by: _____ date ____

      _____   Deliver to: _____

      _____   _____

                                         _____

Send invoice to: _____

                _____

                _____

Item number	Quantity	Description	Unit price
1	2 ea	Olympic-style bench press: Frame 2-1/2 inch square tubing of 11-gauge steel Uprights 49 inches wide and 38 inches high Pad 10 feet wide, 46 inches long, and 16 inches off floor Color of frame, (school color) Upholstery, (school color) Pads made of high-density foam Foot plates with holes so bench can be bolted to floor Safety catch where bar rests: 2-1/2 inches wide, 2 inches deep, and back part 10 inches high, for safety All of frame solid welded for stability	$420
2	10 ea	45-pound Olympic-size plates: All plates machine made for accuracy Edges of plates rounded Color of plates, black Plate style must match existing plates we already have	$ 32

Account name _____   Approved _____

Account number _____   Contact _____

Phone number _____

Ordered by (person initiating requisition):

_____

_____

Figure 2.2 Sample requisition.

allow only previously agreed-upon substitutions.

Should any instructional material come with the equipment? Some equipment is very basic and requires no instructions; more complex equipment should come with an instruction and maintenance manual. The maintenance manual should tell you what to do to keep that piece of equipment working properly for a long time. It should include information on how to order parts from the company if a repair is necessary and a number to call with questions about troubleshooting problems with the equipment.

If you can, order maintenance or replacement parts, like extra cables for pulling machines or extra upholstery, along with the new equipment so you can make simple repairs immediately if you need to. If you do not have those things on hand, when your equipment needs repair you will be at the mercy of the distributor to get the parts to you. This can take several weeks, during which time the apparatus is not usable. Ordering extra parts with the equipment can help alleviate this problem.

EQUIPMENT SPECIFICATIONS

The following section outlines specifics to consider when you are buying new equipment.

Frame

For safety and durability equipment should be made of 2-inch or 2-1/2-inch square steel tubing. Stay away from flimsy or round tubing (usually found in home models) because it might not withstand the heavy use and poundages your athletes will inflict on it. The steel should be of 11-gauge thickness. Thicker than 11 gauge is not necessary, and thinner than 11 gauge is not advised because the price difference is not that great (the larger the number, the thicker the gauge). A practical method of determining steel gauge is to look at the corners of the steel. The rounder the corners, the thicker the steel. If the corners of your equipment are very sharp, you know the tubing is very thin. An 11-gauge tube should have a nice round corner.

A solid piece that requires no assembly is best. Equipment that needs assembly is more likely to work loose. If you cannot move large pieces through the weight room door, some equipment assembly will be required. Measure all entrances before ordering equipment.

All edges should be ground so they are not sharp, and all exposed ends of the equipment should be capped. Any holes drilled through the equipment should be smooth and free of splinters.

Each piece of equipment should have foot holders so it sits solidly on the floor. If it has straight bars as supports and the floor is uneven, the equipment will rock.

Paint

All visible parts of the frame should be painted. A primer is necessary for all painted equipment. The metal should be cleaned before the primer is applied, and one or two coats of paint is enough. Some companies use an electrostatic process (baking the paint on) that is more durable but also more expensive.

Padding

The most durable and comfortable padding is a high-density closed-cell foam. It is extra-spongy and gives good support. Avoid very soft foams (open cell) that do not last long. A 1-inch, high-density closed-cell padding should be enough for most equipment but for areas of high stress (neck, shoulder areas) a 2-inch, high-density closed-cell pad is recommended. The padding should go around the edges of the wood.

Upholstery

Judge upholstery quality by the surface and the mesh behind it. The thicker the surface and the stronger the mesh, the better. Poor upholstery stretches and tears easily. Upholstery should be stapled to the back of the board with staples placed no further than an inch apart. Some companies stitch the corners or seams; this looks nice but is expensive. If upholstery is sewn it should be with nylon thread. All visible open areas, such as the backs of seats, should be covered with upholstery.

Wood

Seats and pads that are covered with upholstery should be made of plywood, not particle board. Birch plywood is the strongest type and does not splinter, but it is quite expensive. All edges and corners of any wood surface should be rounded.

Seats and Pads

For best assembly and aesthetics use T-nut assembly, in which a nut is fixed into the wood where the bolt attaching the wood to the frame is anchored. Use case-hardened bolts when screwing on the T-nuts. Never use wood screws, which quickly come loose.

Pulleys

Pulleys should have ball bearings instead of bushings for longer life and smoother work. If they don't, use high-density, self-lubricating brass bushings. The bigger the pulley (no more than 8 inches in diameter), the smoother the pull. The smoother the pull, the better. The cable should fit snugly in the pulley.

Bushings

Bushings used in pulleys, plate stacks, and other moving parts should be made of low-friction brass with high resistance. These can sometimes be substituted in pulleys for ball bearings, which are even better but are much more expensive.

Rods

Rods on machines should be made of solid cold-hardened steel. Hollow rods are not as sturdy. You can tell them apart by weight; cold-hardened steel rods are much heavier. One-inch rods are very hard to bend and last longer. Thinner, hollow rods can bend, especially during delivery from the dealer to your facility.

Cables, Chains, or Nylon Belts

Machines have one of these three types of attachments moving the weight stack. Chains last longer but create more friction and do not operate as smoothly, and they are considerably more expensive. New equipment may have nylon belts made of Kevlar; these are very long-lasting and create very little friction or noise, but again, they are very expensive. For meeting

both price and efficiency requirements, nylon-coated aircraft cables are the best.

Cables should be fastened together with pressurized fasteners made of lead for resistance. Cables must match pulley grooves.

Hooks

Never use S-hooks to hook handles on the cable; use snap-on hooks for safety. S-hooks are unsafe because they can slip.

Bars

Two things to look at closely regarding bars are the bar's tensile strength and the construction of the sleeves. Tensile strength is the maximum capacity the bar can handle before it bends or breaks. The higher the tensile strength, the better the bar. For heavy lifting a minimum of a 1,000-pound tensile strength is recommended. The sleeves should rotate smoothly and be self-lubricating. For this reason they should have ball bearings or brass bushings.

The power bar is thicker and does not flex as easily as an Olympic bar. It is made to bench, squat, and dead lift heavy loads.

Olympic bars should be flexible but still have a very high tensile strength. Because the Olympic bar is more flexible it is best for use in exercises on the platform (power clean, snatches, jerks). Standard bars should not be used for these exercises because they do not have sleeves that enable the weights to rotate. If the weights cannot rotate, the action can cause wrist and elbow joint injuries. Standard bars can be used for some auxiliary exercises.

Collars

These should be strong and should fasten securely to the bar. The best type is a spin-lock collar that spins on and that you secure by tightening the levers. The poorest are squeeze collars (which are like springs) or those that do not have a tight enough grasp.

Dumbbells

These should be made of cast iron or solid steel. They can be made of one solid piece or several small weight plates fastened together. If they are plate-loaded, they should fasten tightly so the plates do not move. This is usually accomplished by a heavy washer welded at each end. Dumbbells should be well balanced and feel comfortable in the hands. You will find that a knurled handle with a 1-1/4-inch diameter is the most comfortable. For better adaptability, the weight increments should be 2-1/2 pounds from one pair to the next instead of 5 pounds. This means a lot more dumbbells at a higher cost. Cast-iron dumbbells are less expensive than solid-steel ones.

Plates

Plates should be made of cast iron. When first cast, the plates are rough and heavier than their intended weight. The final product should be machine-finished to provide accurate weight and make plate edges smoother. Some plates can vary as much as 2 pounds from the weight indicated on them. Weigh the plates to see if they are accurate. If the weight variance is too high (more than 1/2 pound) reject the plates and have the company replace them. The plate hole should be machine-finished for tighter fit on the bar. All plates should be painted or have another long-lasting finish.

When buying additional plates, try to buy the same brand you already have. Different brands of plates weigh the same but might be different in shape and diameter.

Benches and Racks

These kinds of apparatus need to be adjustable so that any size athlete can use them properly. For example, squat racks should adjust so the bar rests high or low as needed. The seats of all bench-type apparatus should be low enough so the athlete can sit comfortably with feet on the floor. This equipment should also have spotting platforms or safety devices where necessary (see chapter 4, "Weight Room Safety"). Depending on your needs, you may want your equipment to be versatile enough so that athletes can do a variety of exercises on them, especially if your space and budget are limited (e.g., a bench that can change into an incline when you adjust the seat and stands).

EQUIPMENT MAINTENANCE

For longer life and safer use, maintain all equipment in top condition. Check it periodically.

Damage Prevention

To prevent damage to your equipment, follow these guidelines:

- Never leave weights on the bars. After athletes complete the exercises, they should take all weights off the bars. If the weights are left on, especially if the support stands are narrow, the bar will bend.
- Never let athletes drop or throw barbells or dumbbells to the floor. These should be lowered under control. Use bumper plates and rubberized floor mats when athletes do pulling exercises such as the power clean.
- Weight stacks on machines should not be pulled all the way to the top and banged against the pulley, nor should they be dropped abruptly, because the plates might break.
- All weights should be stored on weight racks, not on the floor. Even big weight plates can break, so handle them with care.
- Never let your athletes lie on equipment with their bare skin. Have them wear shirts or use towels to prevent the upholstery from absorbing body oils that make the material deteriorate. This also helps keep the equipment sanitary.

General Maintenance

The following are general guidelines; for more specific directions see the equipment manufacturer's guide. (See also Figure 2.3.)

- Clean upholstery with warm water and mild soap. If it is very dirty or unsanitary, use a disinfectant and water. Avoid habitual use of strong detergents or disinfectants because they remove moisture from the upholstery and can cause it to crack.
- Never use heavy detergent to clean equipment frames. It will erode the paint and encourage rust. Use a sponge dampened with mild soap and water.
- Clean the rods of selectorized equipment with acetone and lubricate them with WD-40 to keep them smooth. Do not use oil or grease unless such use is specified by the manufacturer.
- If cables show any signs of wear (i.e., splintering or shearing) replace them immediately. Healthy cables should be smooth and free of any defects.

Weekly	Monthly	Yearly
Clean upholstery	Clean frames	Replace worn padding
Lubricate rods	Dust chains	Replace worn or bent bars
Check cables	Spray bushings	Replace torn upholstery
Check bolts	Check bar sleeves	Replace bent rods
		Replace broken plates

Figure 2.3   Sample maintenance schedule.

- Keep chains and moving parts free of dust. Wipe the chains with a soft cloth moistened with 30-weight motor oil to keep them working smoothly.
- Check all bolts and moving attachments and tighten them if necessary.
- Lubricate inside the bar sleeves occasionally when you see that the rotation is not very smooth.
- Check the bars for straightness by putting them on the floor and rotating the shaft. If it spins smoothly, the bar is in good shape. If it wobbles, the bar is starting to bend and may need to be replaced.
- If the original foam on benches and other pads has lost its resilience or is too soft, replace it.
- Always use proper selection pins for variable resistance machines as specified by the equipment manufacturer. Do not use nails or rods in place of the correct pins.
- Some maintenance or spare parts are readily available from your local retailer. Other parts may be very specific and you can obtain them only from the manufacturer. See Figure 2.4.

MAKING YOUR OWN EQUIPMENT

Because of budget limitations many coaches and schools rely on their machine or welding shops to make their equipment. I have seen some very good equipment made this way, but I have seen some very poor equipment as well. In those cases I do not believe it was worth the cost and the time. Before you build your own equipment, please be aware of these points.

- Who is responsible if something goes wrong because of an equipment defect—for example, if a weld breaks—and someone is injured? When you buy from a well-known company, it stands behind its product.
- You may see a piece of equipment you like and try to duplicate it. But seldom will the piece turn out exactly the same as the original, especially if it is a machine with several moving parts. On the other hand, it is relatively easy to build a rack or bench press, because these have no complex moving parts (see Figure 2.5). Be sure you have the

Equipment	Place of Purchase
1. Upholstery	Dealer, fabric or upholstery store
2. Selectorized pins	Dealer
3. Cables	Dealer, hardware store, marine store
4. Pulleys	Dealer, hardware store, marine store
5. Bushings and bolts	Dealer, hardware store
6. Plywood	Dealer, lumber supply store
7. Padding	Dealer, fabric or upholstery store
8. Cleaning products	Industrial cleaning supply or drugstore
9. Paint	Dealer, paint supply store

Figure 2.4   Sources of spare parts.

Bench press	Squat rack	Utility bench
Incline press	Power rack	Curl stand
Behind-neck press	Dumbbell rack	Preacher curl
Pulling platform	Dip stand	Chalk stand
Sit-up board	Pull-up stand	Belt rack
Plate storage rack		

Figure 2.5 Equipment you can build.

correct specifications by measuring an existing bench in order to get the job done right.

- Use the best materials available. Do not take shortcuts. Refer to the section on ''Equipment Specifications'' earlier in this chapter.
- Have qualified people do the work. Building weight training equipment involves more than just welding two pieces of metal together. The builder must understand exactly how the equipment works and how it will be used.
- If a piece is built incorrectly, scrap it. Do not hang onto bad equipment just because you have it. Use only properly made equipment.

BARBELLS VERSUS MACHINES

What is the best way to strength train, with barbells or with machines (Table 2.1)? Which produces the best results for athletic competitions? Athletes need more than just general physical fitness; they need strength and power, especially in contact sports such as football or wrestling. Sports like basketball, volleyball, track and field, swimming, and baseball also require strength and power. The combination makes athletes move quicker, jump higher, and run faster. To achieve an optimal level of strength and power, athletes should train with barbells, dumbbells, and machines, doing the majority of the work with barbells. Some exercises are best done with barbells and dumbbells whereas others are better with machines.

Barbell exercises are done using standard bars, Olympic bars, and dumbbells. Different weight plates are added to increase the load.

Machine exercises are done on an apparatus with a system of pulleys that move the weight up and down. It seems like everyone is trying to build exercise machines. Because such a variety of machines is available and new ones are

Table 2.1
Comparison of Barbells and Machines

| | Advantages | |
	Barbells	Machines
Cost	X	
Safety		X
Time efficiency	X	
Technique		X
Beginner athletes		X
Power development	X	
Versatility	X	
Motivation	X	
Muscle isolation		X
Variety	X	
Rehabilitation		X
Space efficiency		X

always coming on the market, I am not able to evaluate them all here.

Advantages of Machines

Isolating Muscles

Machines are excellent for isolating a particular muscle group. Machines can also aid in rehabilitation, such as when an athlete needs to work out and take special care of an injured area. For example, an athlete who has an ankle injury and cannot do a full movement in the lower body can use machines to train the muscles around the ankle and maintain or gain lower body strength. In the case of muscle weaknesses, the athlete can use specific machines to zero in on the affected area. Also, certain muscle groups are better trained on machines—for example, the neck muscles.

For Injured Athletes

Machines are especially useful when your athlete has an injury and you want him or her to continue strength training. For example, an athlete with an ankle injury cannot do squats but can still train the legs by doing leg curls and leg extensions with machines.

Easy to Learn

The exercise techniques for machines are less complicated than some barbell exercises and therefore easier for young and beginning athletes to learn. Beginners are sometimes afraid of handling weights, and machines are a good way of helping them over that fear. After an athlete learns the machine techniques he or she should be able to move on to barbells and dumbbells.

If you do not have the time to teach the techniques of barbell exercises or if you cannot supervise or coach the athletes closely, machines would be best for you.

Safety

Machines are safer than free weights for the simple reason that the weights and bar are an integral part of the machine. This reduces the chances of the athlete slipping and falling, or of the weights shifting. This does not mean that people do not get injured while training with machines. No matter which equipment you use, the best way to prevent injury is to be sure athletes use correct techniques and proper load selection.

Advantages of Barbells

One Size Fits All

The barbell can be manipulated to suit the athlete's personal structure instead of the athlete having to adapt to a machine. The athlete can change hand and foot placement as needed to suit muscle angles and to train certain muscle areas more than others. For example, with barbells the athlete can adjust the hand grip to suit shoulder width and can push the weight according to his or her own arm length.

Even with the many variations and adjustments machines allow (e.g., raising or lowering the seat), machines are still inadequate to serve certain body types. For example, people under 5 feet, 5 inches tall (young athletes and most women athletes), very tall people (basketball players), and large athletes (football linemen) may not be able to use the machines properly.

The angles and mechanics of machines will be very improper for those who do not have an "average"-sized body.

Motivation

It's just plain more fun to handle barbells than to sit at a machine. The athletes literally feel the weight. Actually having the weight on their shoulders and hands and moving the weight themselves makes athletes feel stronger and more in control. Machines do not provide that feeling of handling the weight.

You have heard athletes brag about how much they can bench press or arm curl, but how often do they brag about how much they can lift using a machine? This is in a way unfortunate, because all strength exercises are important and the athlete should be motivated to do them all. No matter what apparatus an athlete uses, the program should be the motivator, not the equipment. But the fact remains that in general athletes prefer barbells.

Variety

Variety keeps the muscle growing and keeps the athletes interested. Barbells offer a greater variety of exercises to keep athletes motivated while still promoting strength gains. Typically, only one exercise can be done on each machine. So either you use a lot of different machines, or, if you are limited to a few basic machines, you find your athletes bored with their workouts.

Muscular Balance

Barbells bring to light any weaknesses or imbalances. For example, the barbell bench press will soon expose a weakness or imbalance. When one side is weaker the other side will do more work, causing the weights to come up unevenly. Recognizing the weakness, you can begin to correct it. Machines tend to camouflage weaknesses and imbalances. As the athletes push or pull on a machine, any weakness or imbalance is compensated for by the stronger side, and because the levers are stationary the weight still goes up evenly. The weaker side does less work, remains weaker, and creates an imbalance.

Power Development

Power outputs are higher with total-body barbell exercises than with machines. Studies have shown that Olympic-style exercises produce more power than any other type of exercise.

Joint Stability

Barbells require the athlete to both support and stabilize the weight while doing the exercise (pushing or pulling), which helps to develop stability in the joint area. Machines handle the stability while the athlete has only to push or pull.

Multijoint Movements

Many barbell exercises train a great variety of muscle groups simultaneously, making them more "complete" exercises. For example, a squat or power clean with a barbell trains many muscles at once—the hamstrings, quads, groin, glutes, calves, and others. Most machines work only one muscle area at a time, so the athlete has to do a series of exercises to get the same results. I strongly believe that the more muscle groups that work together simultaneously, the better the exercise suits athletics.

Costs

Barbells, dumbbells, basic benches, and racks are not as expensive as machines. With a limited budget you can get a more complete facility by buying barbells, and you save on maintenance costs as well. With an adequate budget you can buy barbells and a few specific supplemental machines to suit your needs. Also, because of their weight and the special packing they require, machines generally cost more to ship than barbells and dumbbells do.

Maintenance

You also have to consider the cost of maintenance for the chains, pulleys, cables, and other elements of machines.

Time

We never seem to have enough time to conduct as many exercises or workouts as we would like. Every coach is always looking for ways to maximize the time he or she has available. Barbell exercises save time. Exercises done with barbells can train different areas of the body simultaneously, whereas it would take several different exercises using machines to do the same job. With barbells athletes are able to train more muscle areas and be more productive in the time available.

Organizing Your Program

A well-organized program gets results. As a coach you need to look at the different components of an organized program and implement them for the benefit of the athlete.

WORKING WITH YOUR RESOURCES

Every strength program comes with its own set of challenges. Be innovative to get the most out of your own time, space, and equipment.

Finding the Time for Strength Training

One of the most common difficulties in strength training, especially during the playing season, is scheduling the strength workouts. They are commonly done before school starts, during physical education classes, or after school. If these times cannot be used for any reason, you may find the following suggestions helpful.

Lunch: Use half the lunch period. Make sure athletes train before they eat lunch.

Free period: In many curriculums students have two or more free periods each week to spend pursuing a school activity of their choice. This time could be spent in the weight room.

Before practice: Sometimes there is time between the last class and practice. The athlete can use this time to lift weights. The coach must understand that in this situation the athlete will be somewhat fatigued before practice starts.

During practice: If the athlete has spent insufficient time in the weight room, he or she can do some strength training on the field when time permits. The lifting apparatus can be placed close to the practice field. If no equipment is available the athlete can do push-ups, sit-ups, or manual resistance exercises or can run up steps.

End of practice: If practice starts right after classes, athletes can do strength training after practice.

Weekends: Many states do not allow school activities on weekends. If it is allowed, implement some kind of organized strength training.

Commercial facilities: If all else fails, try to arrange something at a local gym or spa.

Time, Space, and Equipment Considerations

Workouts have to be adapted to the available resources. Following are some situations you might face along with suggestions as to how you can make the best of them. Remember, these are only suggestions; be innovative.

The Weight Room Is Available Every Day With Ample Time

This situation might occur in the off-season, though it is quite unrealistic for most programs. With so much time available you have two main options: Strength train four times a week using a split routine followed by conditioning, or strength train the total body three times a week and use the remaining days for conditioning. Even if your equipment is limited, the abundance of time will make it possible to carry out a variety of core and auxiliary exercises. Do not use classic circuit strength training unless the sport requires muscular endurance.

The Weight Room Is Available Every Day for Short Periods

In this case, the athletes could do a little lifting every day. Divide the workouts into upper body one day and lower body the next (split routine). Because your time is limited your exercises will have to be limited, too. Design the workouts around core exercises that train many muscles simultaneously (multijoint exercises such as the bench press, squats, and power cleans). To make the best use of the time divide the group into two sections each day, with one doing upper-body exercises and the other doing lower-body exercises. Classic circuit strength training will be very helpful in this situation, making it possible for several athletes to train in a short time. Classic circuit training should be used primarily for endurance sports, but with some modifications it can also be used for strength/power sports if it is the only option available. (See chapter 7, ''Classic Circuit Training.'')

The Weight Room Is Available Only a Few Days a Week With Ample Time

Because the athletes can lift only two or three times each week, the total body should be trained at each workout. You have plenty of time, so the athletes will be able to do a variety of core and auxiliary exercises. Again, dividing the group gives you time to help everyone. Do not use classic circuit strength training if you desire maximum strength gains.

The Weight Room Is Available Only a Few Days for Short Periods

This is probably the toughest challenge a program can face. Because the athletes can strength train only two or three times a week, they will have to train the total body at each workout. To take full advantage of the limited time, have half the group start with the upper body while the other half starts with lower body exercises. This keeps the players training, not waiting in line. Athletes should perform mostly multijoint core exercises. Once again, classic circuit training should be used primarily for endurance sports but can also be used for strength/power sports if it is the only option available.

Space and Equipment Are Limited but Time Is Ample

Divide the athletes into groups to come in at different times. The fewer athletes you have in the weight room, the better. Design the program to include core and auxiliary exercises. The particular exercises you use will depend on the equipment you have. Because the equipment is limited some athletes should do upper body exercises while the others do lower body exercises. The idea is for every athlete to have access to some kind of apparatus with little time spent waiting.

Space, Equipment, and Time Are Limited

Classic circuit training is the only option you have with these limitations. Design a circuit based on the available equipment. Start the athletes at different stations and rotate them so they use what you have in the least amount of time. Perform as many core exercises as possible. Reduce the number of sets per exercise to accommodate everyone.

Weight Room Flow

Strength training a large number of athletes in a short time is difficult. The weight room flow (how the athletes move from one apparatus to another) is important and should take full advantage of your circumstances.

The best way to train a large number of athletes is to divide them into smaller groups. Smaller groups are easier to manage, allow more one-on-one coaching, and create better competition within the group. In most cases, have each group start at the same time at different exercises. Ideally the groups should come in at different times, but usually that is not possible. Divide the groups using the following criteria:

The sport: Put athletes involved in the same sport, event, or position together.

Strength level: Divide athletes into similar strength groups so they can spot and encourage each other.

Age, experience: Put older, more experienced athletes in a separate group from younger, less experienced athletes.

The amount and type of equipment you have: The greater the quantity of each piece of equipment you have, the larger the groups can be (e.g., four benches vs. two benches). Free-weight exercises take longer because the weights need to be changed.

Let's look at a typical example you might face. Let's say you have only 45 minutes to train 64 athletes and you have enough equipment for your athletes to perform several exercises. These exercises can include three core exercises (bench, squat, dead lift) and four auxiliary exercises (bicep curls, lat pulldowns, abdominals, and leg curls). First divide the athletes into four groups of 16. Start each group at a different station. The stations are the bench press, the squat, the dead lift, and the auxiliary exercises. The training duration at each station is approximately 11 minutes (45 minutes divided by four stations equals approximately 11 minutes at each station). In that time each athlete might be able to perform 3 to 5 sets of the core exercises. At the end of the 11 minutes each group rotates to the next station. For 16 athletes to train adequately in 11 minutes, each core exercise station should have four apparatus (four benches, four squat racks, four areas to dead lift, and at least one apparatus for each of the four auxiliary exercises).

At the auxiliary exercise station the athlete should be able to perform 2 or 3 sets of each exercise in the 11 minutes. The more equipment available, the more sets the athletes can do in the time allotted. At the end of the 45 minutes each of the athletes will have gone through all four stations, completing the workout. On each workout day start the groups at different stations. Be aware that the group that starts with the auxiliary exercises will pre-fatigue certain muscles before doing the core exercises. See Figure 3.1 for an illustration of this sample flow.

Station 1			
Bench press	Bench press	Bench press	Bench press
X	X	X	X
X	X	X	X
X	X	X	X
X	X	X	X
Station 2			
Squat	Squat	Squat	Squat
X	X	X	X
X	X	X	X
X	X	X	X
X	X	X	X
Station 3			
Dead lift	Dead lift	Dead lift	Dead lift
X	X	X	X
X	X	X	X
X	X	X	X
X	X	X	X
Station 4			
Bicep curl	Lat pull	Abdominals	Leg curl
X	X	X	X
X	X	X	X
X	X	X	X
X	X	X	X

Figure 3.1 Sample flow for training a large group of athletes.

SUPERVISION IN THE WEIGHT ROOM

No matter how organized you are, you alone cannot train hundreds of athletes. Most college-level strength coaches have full- or part-time assistants. In high school, however, if no strength coach is available, you, the sport coach, will need the help of your assistants or other sport coaches. Also, high school strength coaches may need the sport coaches to help supervise the workouts of their teams. The strength coach sets up and administers the program and gets the sport coaches to help with on-the-floor coaching.

The more support you get, the better the athletes will be coached and supervised. Each assisting coach should have a specific duty assigned by the coach in charge. If a coach just hangs around and chats with the players, you are better off without that coach in the weight room. Make sure you and whoever is helping you will actually *coach* in the weight room. Assistants should understand that coaching is as important in strength training as it is in the sport itself.

The weight room should be staffed by qualified personnel at all times. This means the strength coach or sport coaches. Avoid having parents, senior athletes, or others in charge of the program. Do not give the weight room keys to athletes and tell them to go work out. This approach only leads to unwelcome problems like injuries or legal considerations.

When coaches help you in the weight room it is important that they have (a) a good basic knowledge of strength training techniques; (b) a complete understanding of safety-spotting procedures; (c) enthusiasm about the program—they should coach, not just be there; and (d) consistent attendance.

Two or More Coaches

Two systems can be used when several coaches are available to help in the weight room.

Coaching By Exercise Area

Each coach is assigned a specific area to supervise. He or she stays in that area and helps all the athletes doing exercises there. This allows the coach to be in touch with the whole team in one particular area of strength training. If you have two coaches, one could supervise the upper-body exercises and the other the lower-body exercises. With three coaches, one coach supervises the core upper-body exercises, the second the core lower-body exercises, and the third the auxiliary exercises.

Coaching By Groups

Each coach has a specific group of athletes who train at a specific time. He or she takes the group through the entire workout, exercise by exercise, until the workout is complete. When that group is done the coach starts over with another group. For example, if you have 20 athletes working out and two coaches, each coach manages 10 athletes. If you have 60 athletes and three coaches, each coach manages 20 athletes.

One Coach Does It All

If you are the only coach available during workouts, arrange the athletes in small groups and have each group come in at different times. This way you can help each player through each exercise. The size of the squad, the amount of time the athletes have to spend, and the availability of the weight room will determine the number and size of the groups. The worst-case scenario is having a lot of athletes in the weight room at the same time. In this situation you cannot possibly supervise each athlete in each exercise. Therefore, you must concentrate on the core and more complex exercises (power clean, squat, bench, etc.), which require constant supervision.

Coaches' Qualifications

What makes a person qualified to design and implement a strength training program? What should school officials look for when hiring someone or assigning the responsibilities for a strength training program? What will make a sport coach have 100% confidence in the strength coach? These are all valid questions that need to be addressed. I believe the person running the strength program should have the following characteristics: (a) an understanding of the sport, (b) the ability to work with young athletes, (c) knowledge of lifting techniques and safety considerations, (d) knowledge of program design, and (e) a sense of organization. Let's look at who I think is best qualified to run a strength program.

The Certified Strength and Conditioning Specialist

The certified strength and conditioning specialist is probably the best qualified person to run a program. This specialist has passed a very thorough examination given by the National Strength and Conditioning Association and thereby has demonstrated a knowledge of the basic practical and theoretical aspects of strength training.

The Strength Coach

This person has specialized in the field of strength training. As with all coaches, some strength coaches are better than others. They rely on their coaching experiences, their past lifting experiences, and their education.

The Sport Coach

The sport coach's main interest is a particular sport, not exclusively strength training. I know several sport coaches who run very good strength programs, but they also have a real interest in strength training. Because they wanted to do all they could to improve their teams and themselves, they became well qualified to run the program. If you are a sport coach involved with the strength program, learn everything you can about strength training and become as qualified as possible in that field. Increase your knowledge by attending strength clinics, becoming a member of the National Strength and Conditioning Association, and reading the literature published by this association. You should also communicate with other sport coaches about strength training issues and, most importantly, keep up with the development of new equipment, training methods, and formats.

The Weight Lifter

Merely being strong or knowing how to lift weights does not qualify a person to run a strength program. Lifting weights is quite different from strength training athletes. If a weight lifter is your only alternative, make sure that person gets a crash course in understanding the demands of sports, understanding young athletes, and integrating a strength program into sport performance. Of course, this person may do very well if he or she is determined to understand strength training.

RECORD KEEPING

A good record-keeping system is an important part of a well-organized program. Keep records of your athletes' personal bests, workout progress, injuries, body weight, and absences. Having these records readily available makes it easier to determine why an athlete is not progressing as desired (e.g., due to an injury or several absences). A cross-evaluation of several statistics can also tell you why one athlete is progressing faster than another. Having written proof of all this information is essential when you are encouraging athletes to reach new strength levels. It can also help you answer a sport coach's questions about an athlete's progress.

One of the hardest aspects of record keeping is recording all workouts (exercise by exercise, set by set) done by all your athletes. This is an almost impossible task for you to do alone. You will need the athletes' help. You are responsible for getting the recording sheets ready; these show the exercises and the sets and reps of the weight lifted. The athletes do the actual recording. Each athlete should have his or her own recording sheet that shows the workout(s) for the day or week and provides spaces for writing in the weight that was lifted. The athlete fills in the card during the workout and returns it to the coach at the end of the workout.

After the workout is complete, you review the cards to make sure each athlete is making progress. You can even enter the amount of weight you want each athlete to do in the next workout. You can also write in comments that will benefit the athlete. This is very time-consuming, but it really pays off. The athletes see that you have looked at their cards and know that what they write down will be evaluated. This recording of daily workouts also helps each athlete see his or her progress. Athletes do not always remember what they did in previous workouts. The card lets them see what they did last time and what has to be done today, and keeps them on the right track.

	Fall _1988_	Winter _1989_	Fall _1989_	Winter _1990_
Name: _Mark Jones_				
Bench press	210 lb	215	240	240
Squat	305	300	320	340
Power clean	170	185	190	200
Name: _Tom Olson_				
Bench press	160	160	170	185
Squat	254	260	270	280
Power clean	135	135	150	155

Figure 3.2   Chart for tracking strength progress.

What to Record

You may want to use this filing/record-keeping system with your athletes.

Strength Personal Best

Each time the athlete is tested, record the weight on a composite sheet as shown in Figure 3.2. This gives you accurate information on his or her strength progress over the years.

Body Weight Chart

Keep track of athletes' seasonal body weights using a chart similar to Figure 3.2. To record your athletes' daily or weekly body weights, use a chart similar to Figure 3.3.

Attendance Chart

At each workout update an attendance chart so you can see who has been consistent with workouts, especially during the off-season or summer months. You can use a basic chart as shown in Figure 3.4.

Injury Chart

All small or major injuries should be recorded, because they will affect what the athlete can do in the weight room both now and in the future. A simple listing should include the athlete's name, the injury, and how the injury will affect the workout. See Figure 3.5.

Name	Dates				
	9/5	9/6	9/7	9/10	9/11
Marcia Brown	135	135	137	A	137
Paula Pierce	120	121	121	120	121

Note: A = absent

Figure 3.3   Chart for tracking body weight fluctuations.

Name	Dates				
	9/5	9/7	9/9	9/12	9/14
Bill Bower	P	P	A	Sick	P
Tony Morano	P	P	P	P	P

Note: P = present; A = absent

Figure 3.4   Chart for recording attendance.

Name	Date	Injury
Cindy Logan	9/10/89	Sprained ankle No squats 4 weeks
	8/6/90	Sick - missed 1 week

Figure 3.5   Chart for recording injuries.

Workout Progress Chart

Figure 3.6 shows a very basic workout progress chart. You write down the prescribed exercises and the sets and reps to be performed each day. The athlete fills in the spaces to the right with the actual weight performed.

Name: _____

Monday Exercises	Sets x reps	Date: Set 1/2	Set 3/4	Com-ment	Date: Set 1/2	Set 3/4	Com-ment	Date: Set 1/2	Set 3/4	Com-ment	Date: Set 1/2	Set 3/4	Com-ment

Wednesday Exercises	Sets x reps	Date: Set 1/2	Set 3/4	Com-ment	Date: Set 1/2	Set 3/4	Com-ment	Date: Set 1/2	Set 3/4	Com-ment	Date: Set 1/2	Set 3/4	Com-ment

Friday Exercises	Sets x reps	Date: Set 1/2	Set 3/4	Com-ment	Date: Set 1/2	Set 3/4	Com-ment	Date: Set 1/2	Set 3/4	Com-ment	Date: Set 1/2	Set 3/4	Com-ment

Note: Record the weight for each set.

Figure 3.6 Workout progress chart.

DISPLAYING INFORMATION

When I enter a weight room, of course I notice the equipment, but I also notice what the coach displays on the walls to inform and motivate the athletes. I believe this is a very important aspect of a good strength program. It is hard to find time to communicate information to each athlete individually, so you have to post information for athletes to read.

Bulletin Board

Your bulletin boards should be the central source of information and you should update them regularly (Figure 3.7). One bulletin board located outside the weight room should provide limited information when the weight room is closed (e.g., what time the next workout is to be held). A larger bulletin board inside the weight room should hold a greater variety of information. Here are some things you can post:

Workouts

Post the workout schedule for the day, week, or cycle so athletes can see what they are supposed to do today and in the future.

General Information

This pertains to weight room rules and hours, messages, testing dates, and makeup times.

Motivational Material

This can include special articles related to strength, conditioning, nutrition, and substance abuse, among other things. You can also display remarks made by the competition or letters from fans. You may even want a space for the thought for the day, the article of the week, or the player of the week.

Test Results

Posting past test results can inform and motivate the athletes. Test results become more important if they are posted for everyone to see.

Goals

Post goals that were set and agreed to by the athletes. This will remind them of their commit-

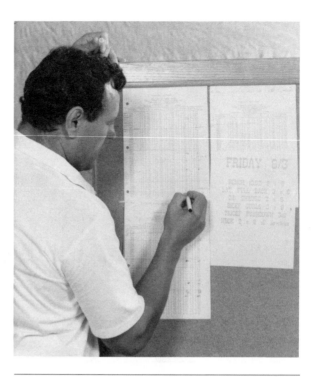

Figure 3.7   Coach updating information on bulletin board.

ment to the program and show each athlete that the rest of the team has made a commitment.

Wall Charts and Boards

You can display a variety of wall charts to inform the athletes.

Exercise Charts

Placing a chart that shows the step-by-step execution of an exercise close to the workout area can help remind the athletes of correct techniques.

Loading the Bar Charts

A simple but informative chart that shows how to get the desired weight will help athletes who have difficulty calculating the exact poundage of a bar with weights (see Figure 3.8).

Record Boards

All strength programs have special ''clubs'' that reward athletes who reach certain exercise levels or goals. You can display these athletes' names and pictures in a special area of the weight room.

Total weight (lb)	Left loading	Bar	Right loading
100 =	Collar 2-1/2 10 10	Bar	10 10 2-1/2 Collar
105 =	Collar 25	Bar	25 Collar
110 =	Collar 2-1/2 25	Bar	25 2-1/2 Collar
115 =	Collar 5 25	Bar	25 5 Collar
120 =	Collar 2-1/2 5 25	Bar	25 5 2-1/2 Collar
125 =	Collar 10 25	Bar	25 10 Collar
130 =	Collar 2-1/2 10 25	Bar	25 10 2-1/2 Collar
135 =	Collar 5 10 25	Bar	25 10 5 Collar
140 =	Collar 2-1/2 5 10 25	Bar	25 10 5 2-1/2 Collar
145 =	Collar 45	Bar	45 Collar
150 =	Collar 2-1/2 45	Bar	45 2-1/2 Collar
155 =	Collar 5 45	Bar	45 5 Collar
160 =	Collar 2-1/2 5 45	Bar	45 5 2-1/2 Collar
165 =	Collar 10 45	Bar	45 10 Collar
170 =	Collar 2-1/2 10 45	Bar	45 10 2-1/2 Collar
175 =	Collar 5 10 45	Bar	45 10 5 Collar
180 =	Collar 2-1/2 5 10 45	Bar	45 10 5 2-1/2 Collar
185 =	Collar 10 10 45	Bar	45 10 10 Collar
190 =	Collar 2-1/2 10 10 45	Bar	45 10 10 2-1/2 Collar
195 =	Collar 25 45	Bar	45 25 Collar
200 =	Collar 2-1/2 25 45	Bar	45 25 2-1/2 Collar
205 =	Collar 5 25 45	Bar	45 25 5 Collar
210 =	Collar 2-1/2 5 25 45	Bar	45 25 5 2-1/2 Collar
215 =	Collar 10 25 45	Bar	45 25 10 Collar
220 =	Collar 2-1/2 10 25 45	Bar	45 25 10 2-1/2 Collar
225 =	Collar 5 10 25 45	Bar	45 25 10 5 Collar
230 =	Collar 2-1/2 5 10 25 45	Bar	45 25 10 5 2-1/2 Collar
235 =	Collar 45 45	Bar	45 45 Collar
240 =	Collar 2-1/2 45 45	Bar	45 45 2-1/2 Collar
245 =	Collar 5 45 45	Bar	45 45 5 Collar
250 =	Collar 2-1/2 5 45 45	Bar	45 45 5 2-1/2 Collar
255 =	Collar 10 45 45	Bar	45 45 10 Collar
260 =	Collar 2-1/2 10 45 45	Bar	45 45 10 2-1/2 Collar
265 =	Collar 5 10 45 45	Bar	45 45 10 5 Collar
270 =	Collar 2-1/2 5 10 45 45	Bar	45 45 10 5 2-1/2 Collar
275 =	Collar 10 10 45 45	Bar	45 45 10 10 Collar
280 =	Collar 2-1/2 10 10 45 45	Bar	45 45 10 10 2-1/2 Collar
285 =	Collar 25 45 45	Bar	45 45 25 Collar
290 =	Collar 2-1/2 25 45 45	Bar	45 45 25 2-1/2 Collar
295 =	Collar 5 25 45 45	Bar	45 45 25 5 Collar
300 =	Collar 2-1/2 5 25 45 45	Bar	45 45 25 5 2-1/2 Collar

a

(Cont.)

Figure 3.8 Chart for loading the bar correctly (a); chart on posterboard, ready to be hung in weight room (b).

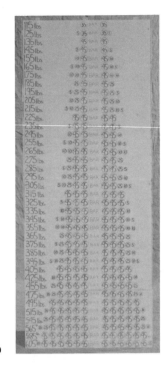

b

Figure 3.8 (Continued)

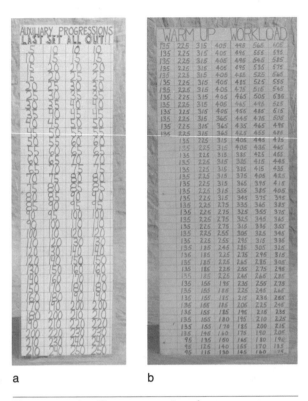

a   b

Figure 3.9 Auxiliary progression chart on posterboard (a); warm-up work loads chart on posterboard (b).

Workout Charts

Post workout charts at different locations around the weight room. Each area the athlete works at should have a copy of the workout posted nearby so he or she knows what exercise to do next. Along with the workout routine, post the necessary charts so the athlete can use the correct weight for each set (Figure 3.9a and b). See chapter 8, "Designing Your Own Program."

Another chart that is handy for weight selection is a percentage chart, with which athletes can quickly tell what percentage of their maximum they are lifting (Figure 3.10).

Visual Aids

A videocassette recorder with monitor and a selection of strength tapes can refresh the athlete in the execution of a particular exercise. You can even videotape an athlete in action and play the tape back for him or her accompanied by your comments.

WORKING WITH OTHERS

Having a nice weight room and good coaches is only part of a successful strength program. In all cases, from small high schools to the college level, you need the help, cooperation, and support of the people around you. Such people include the sport coaches (if you are a strength coach), the athletes, the administration, and even the parents.

Do not expect to get these people's support without appreciating their efforts. Do what you can to make them part of your program. Give them club shirts, invite them to games and to your banquet, and acknowledge them at talks and clinics. This will make them proud to be part of your program and inspire them to continue giving you strong support.

I will now discuss some of these people as well as the things they can do for your strength program.

School Administration

The administration has chosen you as the person to run the strength program; therefore it needs to support you 100%. It should provide the necessary funds to establish a strong program (i.e., facility, equipment, coach's salary). The strength coach, if one is available, is the expert in this area and knows what is needed in the department.

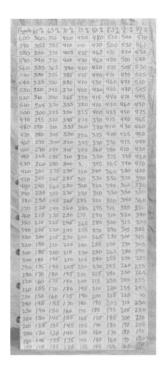

Figure 3.10 Percentage chart on posterboard.

Sport Coaches

A strength coach is of little use to the school if the sport coaches do not involve their athletes in the strength program. The support of the sport coaches can be difficult to get, especially in sports where strength gains are not generally thought to help the athlete. To encourage sport coaches' interest in the strength program, do the following:

- Educate each sport coach about the benefits of strength training as it relates to his or her sport.
- Run an organized strength program. Explain the program in detail to the head coaches whose athletes you will be strength training.
- Understand and take into consideration the sport coaches' philosophy toward training. Usually some compromise can be reached.
- Give the coaches results and comparisons charting the progress of their athletes.
- Show interest by attending the games or competitions.
- Give the coaches strength-related material pertaining to other programs, testimony from successful athletes, or anything else that can help them better understand strength training.

Athletic Trainer

You must work closely with the athletic trainer, if your school has one, and communication between you should be very clear at all times. If an athlete is injured the strength coach should know about the injury. The athlete should strength train the injured area only after the trainer or team doctor has given the OK.

Parents

At the high school level, parents have the final say as to whether an athlete participates in the strength program. Parental involvement can range from getting the athletes to and from school (carpooling) to donating their time, skills, or money. Some parents can help build, maintain, and update the weight room and equipment.

Team Managers

Managers can help keep the weight room clean and organized. They can help with office work, copy and post workouts, keep the bulletin boards up to date, take attendance, collect folders at the end of the workout, and much more. Those few extra hands can make the coach's job easier and allow you to do what you are supposed to do—*coach*.

Janitor

The janitor can take pride in the weight program by keeping the weight room spotless. A clean weight room creates a positive atmosphere. Depending on the particular situation, the janitor may be able to clean the upholstery, lube the machines and chains, and do other general maintenance.

Carpentry and Metal Shop

Much of your equipment, such as benches and bulletin boards, can be built in-house (see chapter 2). Teachers in the shop classes can be very helpful in meeting your equipment needs. In these times of budget cuts, some programs cannot survive without this type of assistance.

Audiovisual Department

Because of all the video technology available today, the knowledge of this department's staff can be of great benefit to you. First, you can direct some of your video purchases through the department, saving you money. Second, the department can lend you equipment or can videotape some of your strength training sessions. If you have or will be buying video equipment, the staff can help you choose it and guide you in maintaining the hardware.

Secretary

A secretary is a vital part of any organization. Your secretary can help by typing and organizing weight room materials (workouts, folders, forms, stats, test results).

Art Department

Both teachers and students can do decorative work for the strength program. They can contribute wall graphics, posters, bulletin board materials, logos, and more.

COACH'S CHECKLIST

Before the start of every workout everything should be ready to go. Referring to this checklist every day may facilitate the task of preparation (Figure 3.11).

1. Are the workouts posted?
2. Are the athletes' recording sheets updated?
3. Was everything the athletes will do today covered during orientation?
4. Is all the equipment ready to go?
5. Is the weight room clean and tidy?
6. Are all coaches present and ready?
7. Is the information board updated?
8. Are my recording sheets and notes ready?

Figure 3.11   Checklist to help coaches prepare for a session.

CHAPTER 4

Weight Room Safety

Strength training is quite safe when properly supervised and controlled. You control your athletes' workouts by planning the sets, reps, and amount of weight they will use. You also provide the best possible supervision. But as Murphy's law states, "If something can go wrong, it will." So you have to do everything in your power to reduce the chance of injury in the weight room. Injuries can occur in the simplest of circumstances at home, at work, and, of course, during strength training. But you can do a number of things to make the weight room safer.

First of all, you can never overemphasize the importance of weight room safety to the athletes. The same seriousness and concentration that applies to all sports, practices, and competitions must apply to strength training as well.

WEIGHT ROOM RULES AND REGULATIONS

Every weight room should have a set of rules and regulations pertaining to safety. Keep these rules posted, and periodically hand them out to the athletes to keep and review. Rules may vary from one weight room to another, but some very basic rules apply to all.

General Rules and Regulations

1. **Train only in the presence of a qualified coach.** An athlete should never strength train in the facility without a coach present, preferably the strength and conditioning coach if the school has one. The weight room should not be open unless a coach is present.
2. **Follow the prescribed workout.** Athletes should do only the workout given by the coach. They should not attempt weights they cannot handle or exercises that have not been prescribed. You can monitor this situation by watching the athletes, counting reps, and checking workout cards.
3. **Maintain proper conduct at all times.** The weight room is no place for horseplay.
4. **Wear proper attire.** The proper attire for strength training is athletic shoes (with laces tied), socks, and shorts and T-shirt or sweats. Athletes should never strength train in street clothes, wearing jewelry, or with articles (e.g., pens and pencils) in pockets.
5. **No eating, drinking, smoking, or chewing.** Workouts are not the time for snacks or chewing tobacco. Athletes can acci-

dentally swallow these substances during an exercise, creating a choking hazard.

6. **No personal stereos with headphones.** Athletes love to listen to music and music is a great motivator, but it should come from a central system. Athletes wearing headphones cannot hear what is going on around them. If someone gives an instruction or tells them to move out of the way, they may not hear and can get hurt.

7. **Help and respect other athletes.** Always help other athletes by spotting. All athletes have the same right to use the weight room, even if some are weaker than others. Let people work out; do not interfere, harass, or interrupt other people doing their workouts. Everyone should use proper language and show respect for others in the room.

8. **No loitering.** Relatives, friends, or fans can distract or confuse athletes working out and should wait outside until workouts are completed. Only athletes who are working out should be in the weight room.

Proper Attire

Proper attire is necessary to maximize the athlete's work and to assure a level of safety.

1. The athlete should wear loose-fitting or stretchy clothes so the body can move freely. This can be shorts or sweatpants. Some athletes prefer sweatpants to keep the bar from rubbing against their thighs during pulling exercises. Shirts should be worn at all times, because bacteria and viruses can be transmitted when bare skin touches the benches. Also, sweat can make the upholstery slick, causing the athlete to shift or slide off. Athletes should remove all jewelry (watches, rings, chains) for workouts.

2. Require athletes to wear good shoes (with laces tied) in the weight room. Several major shoe manufacturers make shoes specifically designed for weight lifting, but good tennis shoes will do the job just fine (Figure 4.1). The shoes should have a firm sole and good heel support to reduce any side movement during the exercise. They should be lightweight and pliable. Typical running shoes have soles that are too soft and that

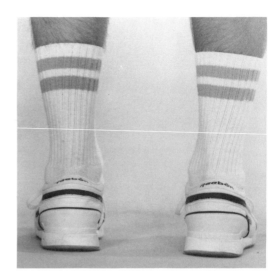

Figure 4.1 Proper shoes for strength training.

can place excessive stress on the ankles when the athlete is supporting weights.

3. There is conflicting evidence concerning the use of lifting belts, but I recommend them. They help keep the back and abdominal area feeling strong and psychologically help the athlete feel more secure. Belts should be strong, able to support the back, and worn tight during the exercise (Figure 4.2). Worn or weak belts should be replaced.

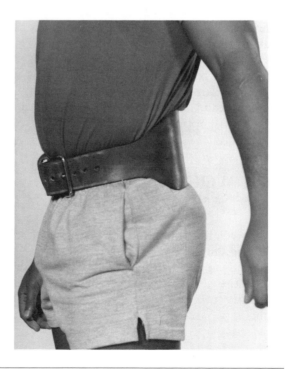

Figure 4.2 Lifting belts should be worn for support.

4. Lifting straps are useful for advanced athletes who handle heavy weights in pulling exercises such as dead lifts and power cleans (Figure 4.3). Straps help the athlete hang onto the bar longer, permitting more repetitions. In certain situations, if straps are not used the athlete's grip gives way before the desired reps are completed. Strength gains then are limited to how long the athlete can hang onto the bar.

Athletes should not overuse straps, however, because overuse may hamper the development of grip strength. To allow proper hand and wrist strength development, do not let very young or inexperienced athletes use straps.

Straps should not be used when the bar is pulled over the head (e.g., in the power snatch). Nor should they be used in warm-ups or with submaximum weights, even by advanced athletes.

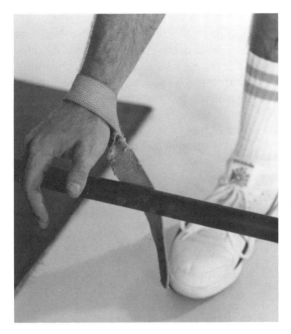

a

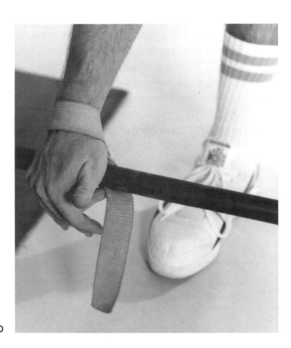

b

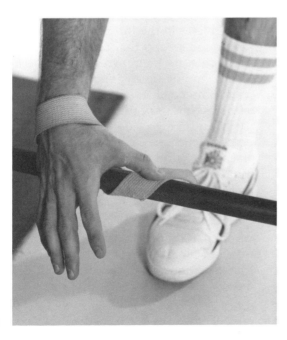

c

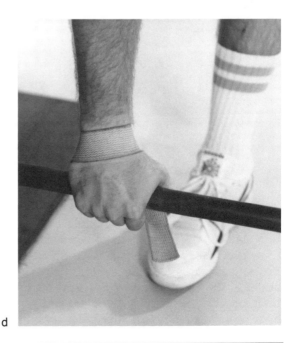

d

Figure 4.3   Proper sequence for using lifting straps.

5. Knee wraps give the knee area extra support to allow the athlete to squat more weight. However, I am opposed to their use for this exercise. I believe they can inhibit knee strength because most of the support is held by the wraps. Athletes need strong knees and knee stability as well as strong quads and hamstrings. Without wraps they can strengthen the stabilizing ligaments, tendons, and muscles in the knee area.

Power lifters use knee wraps because their objective is to lift as much weight as possible, but athletes should be more concerned with their performance on the field, court, or track or in the pool.

6. Chalk (magnesium carbonate) keeps the hands and fingers dry to help athletes maintain a good grip (Figure 4.4). It can also be put on the front or back of a T-shirt where a bar rests if that area is wet from perspiration.

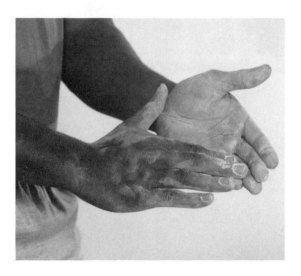

Figure 4.4   When using chalk, cover the whole area.

ORIENTATION

At least once a year, before a new season or off-season program starts, schedule an orientation day (or days) for your athletes. Use this time to explain necessary safety guidelines and proper techniques. This orientation gives new athletes the information they need to make their program safe and productive and serves as a refresher course for the older athletes. I know you are eager to get started on your program, but taking the time to educate your athletes can prevent injuries. Orientation does not stop with those couple of days, however; your athletes need daily reminders of certain points:

- Throughout the program, continue showing athletes the proper techniques of the exercises they will be performing. You can demonstrate them yourself, have an older athlete do them, or show videotapes. Whichever method you choose, the athlete should have a clear mental picture of each exercise before he or she attempts it. The demonstrations should show and explain the procedures step by step. Be patient; athletes cannot learn lifting techniques in a couple of days. The larger the group, the harder it is for you to teach new techniques. Some exercises are harder to teach (and learn) than others (e.g., power clean vs. leg extensions). You need to work with the athletes every day on their lifting techniques. Many basic core and auxiliary exercise techniques are explained in Part III, "Strength Training Exercises," of this book.

- Stress concentration on technique and the importance of keeping one's mind on the workout. Strength training is not a game and can be dangerous if the athletes are not careful and do not concentrate fully.

- Explain in detail the weight room rules, regulations, and procedures. Post this information in the weight room and give it to the athletes in the form of handouts. Help them understand that they must abide by these rules for their own benefit and safety.

- Teach and/or review spotting procedures and techniques. Take the time to show the athletes how spotting is done to make strength training safe. Then have the athletes practice the different techniques with each other under your supervision. Spotting techniques are discussed in more detail later in this chapter.

- Teach and/or review the proper breathing techniques athletes should use while strength training. Breathing techniques are covered later in this chapter and in the exercise techniques sections in Part III of this book.

- Explain to athletes the importance of working within their own limitations—their strength level, their age, and even the equipment. Make them aware of those limitations and instruct them not to go beyond them or try things that are not part of their program. This might be one of the hardest rules for athletes to follow. Trying to outdo teammates can lead to injury. Athletes must work hard not to let their egos get in the way of success.

- Familiarize each athlete with every piece of equipment in the weight room. Explain what each piece of equipment is used for, how it is used, and relevant safety guidelines.
- Explain how to adjust the equipment to suit each individual, how to load and unload the bars, and how to use safety pins in weight stacks.
- Show athletes where the workouts will be posted and explain how to read them.
- Give athletes the training schedule. Let them know who trains at what time and where, so there is no conflict.
- Tell each athlete whom he or she should report to and which coach is responsible for what. If there are several coaches, athletes should know what each coach's responsibilities are.
- Show athletes where to record their workouts and how to keep track of their progress if that is part of your procedures.

SPOTTING TECHNIQUES

All athletes must learn proper spotting techniques and understand the very important role they play in a strength training session. Athletes can take turns spotting each other in pairs or in groups. Spotters should be of similar size and strength as the trainee; a 100-pound athlete might not be able to spot a 400-pound bench press attempt.

A spotter is there if the trainee needs extra help. Sometimes just having a spotter present gives the athlete the confidence to do more in that exercise.

The trainee must understand that the spotter (or spotters) is not there to take over. An athlete who has difficulty finishing a repetition should stay with the bar and continue to try while the spotter(s) assists. The trainee should not give up and turn the bar over to the spotter(s).

Before the Start of the Exercise

The athlete should be concentrating on the exercise. The spotter should check that the correct weight is on the bar and that it is loaded evenly with collars secured. If other spotters are involved, they must make sure they are ready. Spotters should stand where they have a secure position. They should not stand on the equipment itself unless a platform is built onto it for that specific purpose (Figure 4.5).

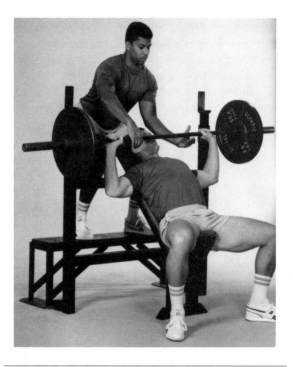

Figure 4.5 Standing on a specially designed platform gives the spotter more leverage.

A spotter must know the exact number of reps the athlete is attempting and how difficult the attempt is for the athlete. Is it a max attempt? Does the athlete think it is going to be very heavy? Knowing this, the spotter will be more aware and ready if the athlete gets distressed.

A spotter also needs to know the athlete's command for help. For example, the athlete can say "Now" to mean the spotter can intervene and help complete the lift. If the athlete says "No," does it mean "Don't touch the bar; I can do it alone" or "I can't do it and need help"? Communication and signals must be very clear between spotter and athlete.

The Lift-Off

Lift-offs are usually done in pressing exercises such as the bench press, incline press, or behind-the-neck press. Some athletes like to have the bar lifted off for them before they start the reps, but most prefer to unrack it themselves. I think it is best if the athlete handles the bar from start to finish, including unracking.

If spotters do help with the lift-off, they and the athlete must clearly understand each other. The trainee has to let the spotters know when to start. It might be a "1, 2, 3, go" order, or a gesture that signals the spotter when to begin. After receiving the signal the spotters use both hands to give a strong lift-off (Figure 4.6). They should not let go of the bar until they are sure the athlete is in complete control. They can even wait for a command from the athlete.

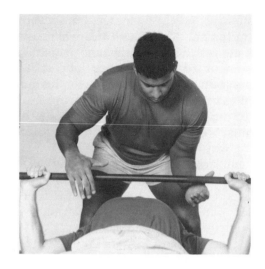

a

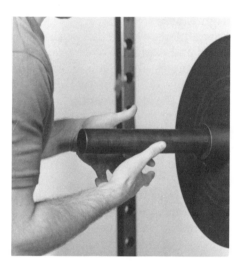

b

Figure 4.7 During the exercise, the spotter's hands should be close to the bar.

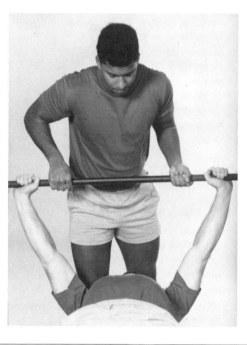

Figure 4.6 When giving a lift-off, the spotter is close and uses both hands.

During the Exercise

No matter what the exercise, spotters must be alert and ready to grab the bar at all times. They must keep their eyes on the bar and the lifter until the set is finished (Figure 4.7a, b).

Spotters should encourage the athlete by saying things like, "Keep it up!" or "You're looking strong!" They can also give coaching tips like, "Keep your back straight" or "Keep your head up." This is very helpful if the spotter knows the athlete's weaknesses and can tell where help is needed, but comments should not be so excessive that they interfere with the athlete's concentration.

If the spotters see the athlete stop in the upward movement, or even slowly come back down, they must assist the athlete immediately (Figure 4.8). If the weight is not very heavy they should help just enough for the athlete to finish the reps of that set. If the weight is too heavy and the athlete cannot move it, the spotters should grab the bar, rack it, and tell the athlete, "That's it, last rep." Here again, good communication between the lifter and spotters is very important.

Pressing exercises usually require only one spotter, positioned as in Figure 4.5. However,

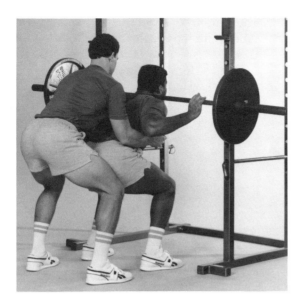

Figure 4.8 The spotter must be ready to assist the athlete immediately. *Note.* Squats with near-maximal loads should be done with three spotters.

with heavy weights, use three spotters, one positioned as in Figure 4.5 and two as in Figure 4.7b. Spotting the squat requires three spotters—two on each side as in Figure 4.7b and one behind as in Figure 4.8.

The End of the Exercise

When the athlete completes the exercise, the spotters should help the athlete rack the bar back on the supports. By this time the athlete is very tired and can use the help. Spotters also help by guiding and directing the bar back onto the rack. Weights should not be slammed back onto the supports because the bar can bounce out.

SAFETY IN BREATHING

During strength training the athlete breathes normally. The athlete takes each repetition individually, breathing between reps. Athletes who hold their breath during the entire set are holding it too long. Doing this can reduce the blood supply to the brain and cause fainting or headaches. This happens often during leg presses, squats, or benches when athletes hold their breath until they finish the whole set.

In most exercises athletes like to hold their breath while they execute the rep, exhaling as the rep is completed. Holding their breath and having full lungs in the initial part of the repetition seems to give them stability and "strength."

Some like to inhale before unracking the bar and hold their breath during the down part. Others unrack the bar and then inhale just before they begin the exercise. Both of these methods are acceptable.

In pushing exercises the athlete should inhale at the top of the lift, then hold the breath during the down part of the movement and part of the upward drive. Shortly after the "sticking point," the athlete should start exhaling to help in the drive upward, then slowly exhale until all the air has been released. The end of the exhalation should coincide with the end of the rep.

In pulling exercises the athlete should inhale just before lifting the bar, hold the breath or inhale during the movement (pulling) part, and exhale slowly during the down part.

SAFETY IN THE FACILITY

In addition to educating the athletes about safety in the weight room, you must provide them a safe environment in the weight room itself. Following these rules will help you keep a safe environment:

1. The weight room must be cleaned regularly, which includes picking up the bars and weights and putting them in their proper places. Lifters should pick up after themselves during the workouts, not just at the end of the day. All objects should be kept off the floor to keep the room clear of obstructions. Personal items such as clothes, gym bags, and other things should be stored in the locker room.
2. The coach should check the equipment regularly (see chapter 2, "Equipment") so that all pieces are in perfect working condition. A piece that is not up to par should not be used, and a sign to that effect should be posted.
3. Equipment should be installed and spaced correctly (see chapter 1, "Your Facility") to reduce the chance of injury or athletes bumping each other. The proper layout will keep the traffic flow smooth and away from the training athletes.

4. On very humid days or when a lot of people are training, the equipment and floor may collect a light film of moisture, causing weights to slip off the bars or athletes to slip on the floor or actually slide off the equipment. Control this with good ventilation, air conditioning, or open windows. Use towels to wipe up the moisture from the floors and equipment if necessary.

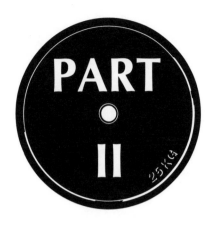

PART

II

BASICS OF
STRENGTH TRAINING

CHAPTER 5

Motivation

Your job as coach is to lead and motivate athletes to reach the highest level of performance possible. On their own, they would probably never get to that point, but you can devise ways to help them. The methods will vary depending on the needs of the program. The athletes' maturity, age, training levels, and success records as well as your own personal philosophy will dictate what motivation you use.

WHY MOTIVATE?

We motivate athletes because we want them to have the desire to participate in and stay with the program. Strength training requires athletes to work constantly at a high level, and without motivation many of them would not stay with it. Motivation makes the program interesting and exciting, creating in the athlete the desire to improve, to excel, and to reach an ultimate goal.

YOUR MOTIVATION

As a coach, your attitude toward strength training will affect the attitudes of your athletes. It's important that you be excited about the program and present a positive image for your athletes to model.

Get Excited

To get others excited about strength training, you and those working with you have to be excited. How can you expect your players to exhibit a positive attitude and enthusiasm if you do not? Enthusiasm is contagious. Let the athletes see genuine enthusiasm in you and your staff. If you try to fake it or treat your position as just a job, your motivation techniques will surely fail, and your strength program will not be successful.

Coach's Image

The strength staff is probably just as involved with the players as their sport coaches are, so it is important that you maintain a respectable image and positive attitude.

Never take your personal problems into the weight room. From the time you come into the facility in the morning until you lock the door at the end of the day, display a positive attitude about the weight room and strength program.

Take a professional approach to your job. Do not discuss a player's failures or problems with any other team member. Treat each player fairly and equally, avoid double standards, and be honest with athletes about their progress.

Because you are involved with the players on a regular basis, it is easy to get close to them, but this can create problems. Some players may get the impression that they can skip a workout without suffering the consequences because they are friends with the coach. Be understanding about players' problems and hear them out, but remain firm if the problems are causing absences or less effort in the workouts. In this way you earn the respect of the players.

In keeping with a professional attitude, do not do your own workouts with the players. The athlete you use as a training partner will be looked on as a favorite by the other team members. Additionally, athletes may feel that you consider your own workout more important than theirs. Furthermore, it is impossible for you to properly coach the athletes if you are busy with your own workout. Do your personal training on your own time.

Most important, you must show a sincere commitment to helping your players. Athletes are adept at spotting the difference between a genuine effort and a phony one.

TYPES OF ATHLETES

I have found that most athletes fall into one of four categories.

Skilled-Motivated

Few athletes fall into this first category. They are the great ones who make your program look terrific. They are wonderful to work with and easily achieve success. These athletes are self-motivated; it takes very little to get them enthusiastic about training.

Unskilled-Motivated

Most of your athletes will fall into this category. They are motivated but not super-talented. Because of their dedication, however, they overcome their physical shortcomings and reach a good level of success. They too are self-motivated. Their own progress often provides enough motivation.

Skilled-Unmotivated

This category is very frustrating, and dealing with these athletes was the hardest thing for me to accept in my early years of coaching. You may have skilled and talented individuals who cannot be motivated. Something in them just does not click. You have to pull out all the stops to get these athletes to reach their potential. This is a true challenge, but not an impossible one. You must be very persistent.

Unskilled-Unmotivated

These athletes do not generally reach a high level of success and may eventually want to drop out of the program. Do not let this happen. Few programs are so blessed that they do not need these athletes. In addition, you have an obligation as a coach to help everyone on the team. You must help them develop physically and mentally to become an asset to the team. You will get great satisfaction from seeing these athletes achieve success because of your persistence.

INTRINSIC AND EXTRINSIC MOTIVATION

Intrinsic motivation (motivation from within) is found in all great athletes. Their self-motivation is based on prestige, recognition, pride, and sometimes even fear of failure. Coaches wish all athletes had this self-motivation.

The motivation you, the coach, provide is called extrinsic motivation (motivation from outside). It usually consists of praise, rewards, and recognition and is used to trigger intrinsic motivation. Because it is temporary and artificial, you do not want the athletes to depend on it. The athlete will succeed only as long as this type of motivation holds his or her interest. Unmotivated athletes need this kind of motivation early in their careers.

WAYS OF MOTIVATING

I have found five basic areas of motivation. If you work on these five areas and implement them into your program, I can almost guarantee your success. Over time, the athletes will *want* to do the workouts instead of feeling forced to do them.

Education

Explain all the "whys" of your program. Tell the athletes why your program is structured the way it is. Describe the benefits they will receive. Without knowing what benefits to expect, athletes may not try as hard. Correlate what is done in the weight room to how it affects the athlete's sport (e.g., squats increase jumping ability). Help them understand that a stronger athlete is less susceptible to injury. Remember, an athlete who asks a question (no matter what type) indicates interest and provides you an opportunity to educate. Keep your own education ongoing. Read training magazines, attend clinics, view videos, get your certification, and continue to expand your own knowledge and expertise. The greater your knowledge base, the more easily you can answer questions, solve problems, and educate and motivate your athletes.

Organized Program

A well-organized program produces results, and positive results are the best motivation an athlete can get. A well-prepared, well-structured program gives athletes confidence and encourages them to give it all they've got. Poor organization (e.g., your being late, not having workouts ready, not planning) puts doubts in the athletes' minds and reduces your program's credibility. Show the athletes you planned thoroughly and did everything you could to create the best program for each athlete. After each workout the athletes should leave the weight room feeling another step closer to reaching their goals.

Recognition

Recognize the efforts each athlete makes. You can do this every day with a small compliment or a pat on the back. Let the athlete know that you are aware he or she is trying hard. A few simple words to acknowledge something achieved in a previous exercise or workout can really mean a lot to the athlete. Showing that you are keeping track of their individual progress makes each athlete try harder. You can show further recognition by giving T-shirts or awards, placing reports in the school newspaper, and making general announcements for all to hear. In team sports, however, try not to overemphasize one individual but recognize instead the whole team or special groups.

Individualized Workouts

All athletes are different and progress at their own pace. Some are more gifted and get stronger before others do. Design a program that will help each athlete get the most out of himself or herself. Use the information given in chapter 8, "Designing Your Own Program," to help you design individual workouts.

Some coaches make the mistake of generalizing the workouts, making everyone lift the same amount of weight and do the same exercises over and over again. In this situation some athletes are undertraining and others are overtraining. Both cases make athletes lose interest in the program and reduce their performance. Along with selecting the right intensity, you and each athlete must set individual goals. I talk more about this in the next section.

Positive Environment

Athletes will benefit from being in a positive environment that is conducive to training. Therefore, follow these guidelines:

Make sure the weight room is clean.

Have unusable equipment repaired as soon as possible.

Get as much equipment of the highest quality as your budget permits.

Paint the equipment and the weight room in your school's colors.

Dress up the weight room walls with team logos, charts, a record board, and slogans.

Play music the athletes like.

Update the record board and awards announcements as soon as you can.

Use the bulletin board to display inspirational stories, pictures of the athletes, articles of interest, and anything else that will help the athletes work harder.

GOAL SETTING

Everyone who aspires to greater heights sets long-term and short-term goals. Together, you, the athlete, and the team must set goals and design a program to reach them. Having a specific weight to lift and a plan to reach that weight is very motivational to the athlete. You can also set goals for attendance, body weight, or eating habits, all of which ultimately affect an athlete's progress.

Guidelines

Follow these guidelines in your goal setting.

- Let the athlete have a voice in setting his or her own goals. Meet with each individual, reach an agreement, and put it on paper for both of you to sign.
- Look at the past and analyze what the athlete has achieved. Consider age, training level, work habits, physical limitations, and past injuries before setting the goals.
- Make the goals challenging but attainable. Do not set goals you know the athlete cannot achieve—that is counterproductive. Goals that are too easy, however, make the rewards meaningless. Help the athlete acknowledge his or her talents and shortcomings and understand the goals you agree on.
- Set long-term and short-term goals. For example, the long-term goal may be performing a desired weight at the end of a training cycle, whereas the short-term goal may be specific week-by-week progress to reach that performance. Athletes can also set long-term goals for two or three years down the road (e.g., the athlete's senior year), and short-term goals for each training cycle until that time. When the ultimate (long-term) goal is broken down into stages (short-term goals), it is easier to attain.
- If unforeseen situations arise (e.g., injuries), reevaluate the goals. Do not continue on the path set before the situation occurred. Reset goals (e.g., rehabilitate the injured area).
- Make the goals specific and measurable. This is quite easy in strength training. The goal can be a specific amount of weight for a designated number of reps in a particular exercise (e.g., 300 lbs bench press for a single rep). Do not set "do what you can do" goals because those provide nothing tangible for the athlete to look forward to. Assess the athlete's progress periodically by testing him or her.
- Set up a game plan as to how the athlete will achieve the goals. Specify the number of workouts and the number of weeks or months needed to reach the goals. Make it clear to the athlete what must be done and the amount of work that is necessary.

What Not to Do

Never embarrass an athlete in any way. Discipline, of course, is sometimes necessary, but do not use humiliation. Negative peer pressure can also be very dangerous. Talk to each athlete privately, not in front of his or her peers. Do not use trickery to get things done; be honest with the athletes.

PLAYING THE NUMBERS GAME

Strength training is a numbers game. Use these numbers to your advantage to get the athletes to perform at higher levels. Post the results of testing for all to see. This creates competition—athletes do not like to be outdone by their friends. Athletes who know what the others have done will put more into their workouts to catch up to or surpass their teammates.

Get in the habit of recording the workouts, and show the athletes what they have done in the past in comparison to the current results. The numbers will speak for themselves, giving the athlete concrete evidence of his or her progress.

Keep in mind, however, that in the numbers game, *progress* is important, not the numbers themselves. For example, some athletes might not be genetically gifted and might never lift a lot of weight, but if they make constant progress, they are getting better, and that is what training is all about.

Be careful not to put too much emphasis on actual numbers. You are training young athletes, not weight lifters. Too much emphasis on numbers might put pressure on athletes to use steroids. If this happens, you have lost it all.

Strength Training Principles

Many coaches who watch weight lifting competitions on television or read muscle magazines are convinced that weight training is not for their athletes. Although competitive weight lifting and strength training do share some similarities, the purpose and results of each are greatly different. The object of strength training is to *reduce injuries and improve sport performance*, not to make competitive weight lifters out of athletes.

Once coaches understand the differences, they can be encouraged to add strength training to their programs and can soon reap the benefits—namely, faster, stronger, more powerful athletes and winning teams. Furthermore, they are delighted to find that their athletes do not look "bulky" or "nonathletic."

In strength training for sports, I have found it best to look at all three competitive weight lifting areas—Olympic lifting, power lifting, and bodybuilding—and use what best suits your sport. All three areas have some good concepts, exercises, and philosophies of training. Using a combination of the three is better than going all in one direction. You might take something like the power clean from Olympic lifting because the explosive movements help generate power. You might take the squat and bench press from power lifting because they are basic strength exercises that add mass and bulk. You might also look at concepts of bodybuilding in auxiliary work to strengthen antagonistic muscles and isolate specific muscle areas.

OVERLOAD PRINCIPLE

For muscles to get stronger they have to be overloaded. Overloading means putting stress (an amount of weight) on the muscle greater than what it is accustomed to. As the muscle adapts to greater levels of stress, the amount of weight that constitutes an overload must be increased. When the muscle is stressed slowly and systematically, it will respond positively and become stronger. On the other hand, sudden large increases in resistance should be avoided, for if the stress is too great the muscle will react negatively with injury or overtraining. The athlete should use realistic increments when increasing the work load from one workout to the next. For example, if the athlete can bench press 200 pounds now, after a couple of workouts the 200 pounds will become easier (the muscles will have adapted to the 200-lb stress). Then the athlete may be able to handle 205 pounds. When the muscle has adapted to the 205 pounds, the athlete can increase the weight again. When the muscles have become accustomed to new overloads, the athlete can perform his or her sport activity more efficiently; faster; and with more strength, greater force, and more endurance.

To increase strength, the athlete must train with relatively heavy loads. Underloaded resistance (below what the muscle normally encounters) will not result in strength increases. A perfect example of underloaded resistance occurs in push-ups. At first the athlete gains strength, but as the muscles get used to the stress (the body weight), no further strength gains are realized. But if resistance is increased (e.g., by a weight plate placed on the athlete's back), strength will increase.

Resistance should be increased throughout the course of the program as the muscles gain in strength and endurance. For this reason the overload principle has been modified to what is called the principle of progressive resistance.

PROGRESSIVE RESISTANCE

Now we know that muscles need an overload to get stronger, but how much should this overload be? Should an athlete lift as much as he or she can in the first workout? In each workout? Progressive resistance involves increasing the weight gradually as the body gets used to the new stress. Start by assigning very realistic weights, then gradually make small increases. Nothing is worse for athletes than continually failing because weight progressions are not sensible. If the athlete can do 200 pounds in the bench press one day, then asking him or her to go to 210 pounds at the next workout is realistic. If you see that 200 pounds is difficult, then you might go to just 205 pounds next time. You must ensure that the athlete can complete all the sets and repetitions. As long as the resistance is increased, the athlete will be gaining strength. Research shows that the total number of repetitions the athlete does may be a secondary consideration in terms of strength development. The most important factor seems to be the use of relatively heavy resistance and near-maximum effort.

PYRAMID SYSTEM

The pyramid system is the most widely used training method for increasing strength. In a pyramid system the athlete performs several sets, starting with light weights and many reps, and increases the weight with each set while reducing the number of reps (Table 6.1). There are many variations to the pyramid system but all have these basic characteristics: multiple sets per exercise, increases in weight, and decreases in the number of repetitions.

Table 6.1
Sample Pyramid Routines

Sample A	Sample B	Sample C
95 × 10	95 × 10	135 × 10
105 × 8	105 × 10	185 × 8
115 × 5	115 × 8	225 × 5
125 × 5	125 × 8	245 × 3
140 × 3	140 × 8	275 × 2
	160 × 5	300 × 1

There is no set formula for setting up a pyramid routine. As long as the weight increases progressively, the reps decrease, and the athlete ends at the desired work load, you are headed in the right direction. It is still a pyramid even if the reps stay the same (e.g., 5 × 5) but the weight increases. The sets and reps do not necessarily need to end with a single in a pyramid routine.

Double Pyramids

In the double pyramid the athlete reaches the top set and then comes back down and does the other sets with less weight (Table 6.2).

Table 6.2
Sample Double Pyramid Routines

Sample A	Sample B
95 × 10	135 × 10
105 × 8	185 × 8
115 × 5	225 × 5
125 × 5	275 × 3
140 × 5	300 × 1
115 × 8	250 × 5
105 × 8	200 × 10

These extra few sets allow more muscle hypertrophy (see section on hypertrophy in this chapter). This method can lead to burnout or overtraining if used incorrectly. Coming back down from heavy sets and doing several more places additional stress on the body, and the athlete needs more time to recuperate.

SPECIFICITY

Specificity in strength training means performing exercises that create strength and power in the specific muscles used in the athlete's sport. This means athletes follow guidelines and use training exercises that simulate the same major movements and energy they need in their sport performance. Metabolic specificity dictates the number of sets, reps, and load used. Biomechanical specificity determines which exercises are used.

Metabolic Specificity

Metabolic specificity refers to how sets, reps, and load are integrated to simulate the physical demands of the sport—either muscular strength/power or muscular endurance. As a coach you must first analyze a sport to determine which is needed. Sports requiring short bursts of activity with some recovery, such as football, track, basketball, and baseball, require muscular strength/power. Athletes gain muscular strength/power by doing exercises at near-maximum loads with few repetitions.

If the sport requires a long, sustained effort and provides little or no chance for recuperation, as in distance running, rowing, racket sports, and wrestling, the athlete should train for muscular endurance by doing exercises with lighter loads, more repetitions, and less recovery.

Biomechanical Specificity

Biomechanical specificity refers to strength training exercises with movement patterns similar to the ones the athlete uses in the sport. Again, as a coach you must study the sport activity to identify which muscle groups play a prime role in it (Figure 6.1). In simulating these movements, it is important that you note the joint angle used in the particular motion. For example, a football linebacker should bench press to develop the muscles used in tackling and blocking. A wrestler should do arm curls and other pulling exercises because of the pulling movements that are very dominant in wrestling. A shot-putter uses a pushing motion and should incorporate exercises that extend the hips, legs, shoulders, and arms.

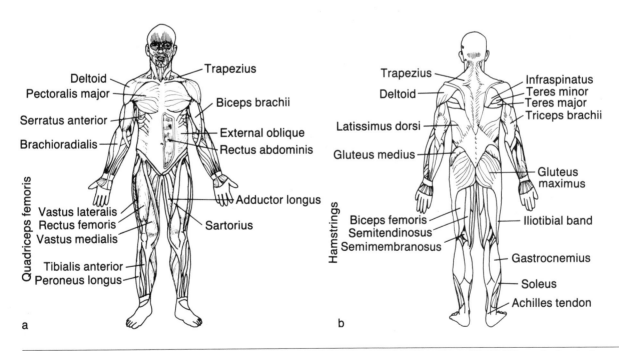

Figure 6.1 Muscles of the human body. Front view (a) and back view (b). *Note*: From *Health/Fitness Instructor's Handbook* (pp. 40-41) by E.T. Howley & B.D. Franks, 1986, Champaign, IL: Human Kinetics. Copyright 1986 by E.T. Howley & B.D. Franks. Adapted by permission.

INTENSITY

Intensity is the amount of tension or stress placed on a muscle. It is determined primarily by the amount of weight used but is also affected by the number of sets and reps, the rest intervals, and the duration of the workout. In this text I use intensity most often to refer to the amount of weight.

What is intense for one person may be easy for another. In strength training intensity is regulated by a percentage of an athlete's personal best. This makes workouts more accurate and more individualized.

For example, say an athlete has a personal best (1RM) of 400 pounds, and today's workout demands 80% intensity for a predetermined number of repetitions. For this workout the athlete will use 320 pounds (80% of 400 lb = 320). If the next workout demands 90%, the amount of weight will be 360 pounds (90% of 400 lb = 360).

You can also differentiate intensity by labeling loads heavy, medium, or light. These terms are also relative. What was heavy to an athlete last month may be light today, and what was light at the end of a cycle might be heavy at the start of a new cycle. When correlating a percentage to heavy, medium, or light, use the following guidelines:

Heavy: 90%–100% effort

Medium: 80%–89% effort

Light: 60%–79% effort

The intensity or actual weight used relates to the time of the cycle. For example, the athlete may have a 400-pound 1RM in the squat. Obviously, when an athlete starts a new cycle, this will be too much weight to handle. Let's assume all the athlete can handle the first week is 250 pounds × 5. This automatically becomes a 100% (heavy) effort at that time. In the next workout the athlete will work at a medium intensity, which might be 225 pounds for the last set. For the next heavy workout, the athlete might do 270 pounds, which is now the new 100% effort; therefore, the next medium workout will be based on 270 pounds. The athlete's goal will be to beat the 400-pound 1RM at the end of the cycle.

VOLUME

In reference to exercises, sets, and reps, volume refers to how many, not how heavy. A high-volume workout means performing many exercises with many sets and reps. Low volume means doing fewer exercises, sets, and reps. To get stronger the athlete needs not only to lift heavier weights but also to increase the volume (more sets, reps, and exercises) as his or her training progresses.

Early in a young athlete's training, he or she gains strength by increasing the volume of the workouts and maintaining a fairly low intensity. As the athlete becomes more accustomed to strength training and his or her body gets used to the stress, the intensity and the volume of the workouts are increased. The advanced athlete does more sets, reps, and exercises at a higher intensity.

For maximum strength/power gains the volume must be kept moderate so the athlete can handle near-maximum weights as required. But for muscular endurance, keep the volume high while keeping the intensity submaximum.

FREQUENCY

Frequency is simply how often the athlete trains within a particular time period. It refers to the number of times the athlete trains each day, each week, or within a cycle. For example, an athlete training once a day three times a week has a frequency of three workouts a week. If the athlete is training once a day four times a week for 10 weeks, the frequency is 40 times for that cycle. Frequency must be regulated and workouts spaced out evenly over the training period. Working out five times one week, then none the next week does not produce good results.

HYPERTROPHY

Hypertrophy is the enlargement of muscle that results from strength training. For years this was attributed solely to an increase in the diameter of the muscle fiber. More recently, though, evidence has attributed increases in muscle size to an increase in the number of fibers (hyperplasia).

But whether by increased fiber diameter or increased fiber number, bigger muscles are not always stronger muscles. There is a *big* difference between strength training and bodybuilder (size-oriented) training. Having big muscles does not necessarily mean a person has great strength; nor are significant increases in strength always accompanied by significant increases in muscle size. In the early stages of training significant increases in muscle size occur. But after an individual has developed a certain muscular size, he or she can gain further strength increases with much smaller gains in muscular size.

An athlete who has to gain weight (muscle mass only, not fat) needs additional hypertrophy training to develop that extra muscle mass. He or she can best accomplish this by first doing the regular workout, then doing extra work. The extra work can include down sets or a variety of auxiliary exercises such as arm curls, shoulder presses, and leg extensions; you may also wish to add another workout each week. Combining the regular workout with additional hypertrophy work without overtraining the athlete will result in faster gains of muscle mass.

Each individual has a different genetic potential for the amount of hypertrophy and strength he or she can gain. Some athletes have to do more work than others to reach the same level. Some may never get to a certain level no matter how much training they do because of their genetic limitations.

NEGATIVE AND POSITIVE TRAINING

In weight training, when the athlete lowers the bar he or she is performing negative work, whereas raising the bar is positive work. In both situations the muscle contracts; therefore, both are important in the development of strength. When the weight is lowered, the muscle is allowed to lengthen while it maintains tension. This is called eccentric contraction or negative resistance. The muscle acts as a stopping mechanism, controlling the movement of the resistance. When the athlete is pushing or pulling

the force the muscle contracts, and the action is called concentric contraction. It is important that the athlete control downward and upward motion in all exercises. For example, in the bench press the athlete should lower the bar slowly instead of "bouncing" it off the chest. In the squat the athlete should lower to a position where thighs are parallel to the floor, momentarily stop, and then push up. If the bar is lowered too fast and it bounces at the bottom, there is no negative contraction in the exercise.

I do not recommend that athletes do negative work exclusively. Doing a lot of negative training can damage muscle tissue, and an athlete will have a hard time recuperating from the workout. It has been shown that when a person engages in heavy negative training, the muscle's ability to handle eccentric work increases, but increases in the ability to handle concentric (positive) loads are limited. Because most movements in athletics are positive (involving extension of body limbs), excessive negative work is not a good idea for training athletes. Always have athletes work both the positive and negative parts of an exercise. On occasion they can perform some extra negative resistance as a variation, but this should be done sparingly.

To perform negative resistance training, the athlete should handle weights heavier than the ones used in the workout—usually 10% to 15% heavier. For example, an athlete who can bench 300 pounds might use 330 pounds for negative repetitions. The athlete should perform these repetitions after completing the prescribed sets and reps. The partner helps raise the weight (positive part), then the athlete tries to lower the weight alone in a very controlled manner under the close supervision of his or her spotter(s).

MUSCLE FATIGUE

Muscle fatigue is a by-product of hard training. A muscle has to be restored before it can be trained again. Constant muscle fatigue is a sign of overtraining. As the athlete improves his or her fitness and strength level, muscle fatigue will be reduced substantially. You can implement principles that will help athletes minimize muscle fatigue and increase muscle performance. Instruct them to follow these guidelines to combat muscle fatigue:

- Allow adequate rest. Getting the right amount of rest during workouts, between workouts, and between training cycles is of utmost importance to minimize muscle fatigue.
- Insure proper nutrition. The muscle must be well nourished because nourishment is an integral part of muscle growth and recuperation. Eating a balanced diet helps the muscle recuperate faster.
- Get enough sleep. Athletes need good sleep; during sleep the muscle recuperates tremendously. Adequate sleep is no less than eight hours a night; many athletes will require more than this. Lack of adequate sleep will affect an athlete's performance.
- Use restoration methods. Several studies show that massage is a very important restoration factor in combating muscle fatigue. Massage relaxes the person, manipulates the muscle area, and accelerates the recovery process. It can be done by hand or in a whirlpool or shower. Steam baths and saunas are also good restorers.
- Do a cool-down. At the end of the activity the athlete must cool down with easy exercises (e.g., jogging) and flexibility exercises. This restores some of the athlete's energy, stretches the muscles, and helps the athlete prepare for the next session.

MUSCULAR SORENESS

The precise cause of muscular soreness is a mystery. We do know there are two kinds of muscular soreness. Acute soreness occurs during or immediately after the workout. It stops when the person stops working out that day. Delayed soreness appears 24 to 48 hours after the workout and can last several days, depending on the fitness level of the person and the amount of work done.

In weight training it is believed that soreness occurs when the muscle is forced to contract eccentrically. For example, lowering the bar in a bench press creates more muscular soreness than pushing the bar up. Another theory is that more muscle fibers are working when the bar is pushed up than when it is lowered. For this reason we must be very careful about athletes doing excessive negatives.

Muscular soreness varies with the athlete's training level. A person who has just started a new training cycle or who is a novice will get sore. But as the person gets stronger and his or her body gets accustomed to the training, there is a lot less soreness.

Muscular soreness also varies with the amount of work done. A person doing a lot of exercises at a high intensity will experience accentuated soreness.

When a person changes exercises, muscular soreness occurs. The new exercises place new stresses on the body, and the body has to become accustomed to the new stress before the soreness ceases.

OVERTRAINING

Overtraining (also referred to as training rut or getting stale) is a condition in which the athlete reaches a plateau, experiences a drop in performance, or both over a period of time. Failure to use proper training principles and procedures is the cause of this very common problem.

How many times have you heard people say, ''If this much work is good, then twice as much should be really good,'' or, ''If I feel tired, I must not be in good shape, so I'd better do more work''? You seldom hear, ''Let's rest today so we can work harder tomorrow.'' Hard work *is* the key to success, but it must be accompanied by rest.

If the body is trained correctly it adapts to stress and becomes stronger. Trained incorrectly, it cannot adapt, becomes weaker, and breaks down. If the athlete works the muscle to failure (exhaustion) too often without enough rest between workouts, the athlete is overtraining. Fatigue and musclar soreness operate as warning devices, so athletes must listen to their bodies.

Observable Signs of Overtraining

The athlete and you should always be on the lookout for signs of overtraining. These are some common signs and the sequence in which they often appear.

The athlete reaches a plateau and cannot continue making progress.

The weights that the athlete once handled quite easily start to feel much heavier.

The athlete feels more fatigue than usual.

The muscles become very sore, more so than they usually do following hard workouts.

The amount of weight the athlete can lift actually decreases.

The athlete does not complete the workouts.

The athlete becomes depressed because he or she is not getting better.

The athlete loses motivation and develops an ''I don't care'' attitude.

Body weight decreases along with loss of appetite.

The body has lowered resistance to headaches, fever blisters, and colds and other illnesses.

The athlete does not sleep well at night.

The athlete experiences an increase in anxiety.

The athlete experiences a decline in performance outside the weight room, such as a drop in academic standing or relationship problems.

Injuries such as pulled ligaments or muscles begin to occur. The muscles are just too fatigued to sustain the amount of stress the athlete is placing on them.

Clinical Signs of Overtraining

These signs are more difficult to detect and monitor. If you suspect the athlete is overtraining, however, you can try to use these methods of detection for a few days. A daily pulse and weight check can tell you if the person is overtraining. The pulse beat rises and the body weight decreases. Have the athlete take his or her pulse on first rising in the morning. You can check the weight during the school day but do so at the same time each day.

A rise in blood pressure is also a good indicator of overtraining. The body is not able to recuperate fast enough and the person's blood pressure rises. To correctly monitor blood pressure, take it on a regular basis at approximately the same time each day.

Avoiding Overtraining

The key to avoiding overtraining is to ensure that athletes train correctly. Athletes and coaches should follow these basic guidelines.

- Do not do too much too soon; that will result in a quick burnout. In a classic example of overtraining, athletes get really gung ho and work, work, work without planning. At first they get great results, which are a positive reinforcement that makes them work even harder. But all of a sudden, fatigue catches up. Recuperating from the overtraining will take days or weeks of reduced training. All that excessive work done in the beginning has gone to waste.

- Workouts must be planned and organized with a good selection of exercises and proper numbers of sets and reps, following a progression that leads to the desired goals.

- The workouts need variety. Many athletes find it difficult to change their routines. They like to start with the same exercises and do the same workout day after day. To provide the greatest benefits, the workouts need periodic changes in the type of exercises performed; order of exercises, sets, and reps; and intensity. Variety promotes muscle strength and growth.

- When making changes in the workout the athlete should not increase the volume *and* intensity at the same time. If the volume is increased, the intensity must be decreased. If the intensity is increased, the volume must be decreased. Only advanced athletes can handle simultaneous increases in volume and intensity.

- Athletes must allow enough rest from one workout to the next. Muscles need to recuperate, usually 48 to 72 hours, before they are trained again.

- Athletes should take good overall care of their bodies. They need more sleep than the average person because they are doing more work and putting more physical stress on their bodies. They should eat good food that is high in nutritional value. You cannot feed the body junk and expect it to perform at a championship level.

- Workouts should be individualized. If all athletes are doing the same exercises, each should be working at his or her own pace using weights he or she is capable of using. Often coaches designate a certain weight that every athlete has to lift. This causes some athletes to undertrain, because they are strong enough to do more. It makes others overtrain because they are not strong enough to handle that much. The athlete should use as much weight as he or she is capable of lifting within a guided program structured to help the athlete reach his or her particular goals.

Recovery From Overtraining

The best possible way athletes can recover from overtraining is with *more rest* and *less work*. You must never tell these athletes to work harder or that they are not trying hard enough. They are already working too hard. They should instead increase their rest, relaxation time, food intake, and sleep. Never confuse ''laziness'' with overtraining.

You can correct a mild case of overtraining by lowering the workout intensity and adding more rest to the athlete's program. Overtraining that is not discovered until very late can be more severe, and it may take days for the athlete to get out of the rut. You may have to excuse the athlete from some practices or substantially reduce the workload over the time it takes him or her to recuperate. The longer overtraining has been going on, the longer it takes for the athlete to begin to feel fresh and for the body to respond again. As the athlete shows he or she is coming out of the overtraining, you can *slowly* begin to increase the intensity of workouts.

Changing the intensity, the number of sets and reps, and the order of exercise also helps the athlete recover from overtraining. Many times signs of overtraining occur not necessarily because the athlete's body is fatigued, but because he or she does the same thing over and over again. The muscles get used to the same workout day after day, and the routine no longer promotes positive strength adaptation.

OTHER CONSIDERATIONS

There are several other factors to be considered in conjunction with strength training. Athletes are often misinformed concerning various topics, so you need to provide them with correct information.

Athletes in Weight Lifting Competition

Many athletes who participate in sports also compete in power lifting, bodybuilding, or Olympic lifting to improve their strength. But the athlete should do this only in the off-season and with the goal of improving in his or her chosen sport. Competitions can be useful for motivation, especially for young athletes. But the athlete should be very careful not to overemphasize the weight lifting competition. Because of the type of training necessary to be a truly competitive weight lifter, athletes can easily get carried away by the competition and do more weight training at the expense of other physical areas (speed, power, conditioning, flexibility). The athlete might also limit exercises by doing only those that will improve weight lifting competition performance, ignoring the original goal of strengthening the total body for his or her sport. The athlete should perform a variety of exercises without placing too much emphasis in one area, which can cause the other areas to become weaker or imbalanced.

Athletes who do compete in weight lifting should continue exercises that are specific to the sport, as well as those that emphasize flexibility, speed training, and conditioning. They should understand that their performance in weight lifting competitions may suffer a little, but they will be better prepared for their main sport.

The Bench Press Syndrome

This term applies to those whose main, and often only, goal is improving their bench press. They have the common misperception that if they can bench press more weight they are becoming stronger, better athletes. In fact, bench press ability is only a small indication of total-body strength. It does not measure lower-body strength or determine how fast and explosive an athlete is.

Like competitive lifters, athletes can get carried away in their obsession with the bench press and eliminate exercises specific to their sports. As a result, performance in their sport declines. When this kind of attitude reigns in the weight room, the entire team can suffer.

Even more important to understand is that an overemphasis on the bench press creates serious muscular imbalances and increases the chance of injury. This is noticeable as an athlete's shoulders begin curving inward toward the chest because the chest muscles are much stronger than the upper-back muscles.

Max Attempts

Just as there are athletes who are obsessed with the bench press, some athletes are obsessed with max attempts (doing all-out single repetitions). They are under the impression that the amount a person can lift for one repetition is the only indication of strength. They feel they have to max out each time they train. Max attempts at every workout leads only to over-training, burnout, and injuries.

Doing ''singles'' is not training, and it does not indicate athletic ability. Doing the workout with the proper sets and reps, with proper progressive resistance, and following the principles of overload is what actually makes an athlete stronger.

CHAPTER 7

Classic Circuit Training

Classic circuit strength training, often referred to as circuit weight training or CWT, consists of a number of exercise stations arranged to allow athletes to rotate quickly from one to another until they have completed the entire workout. The stations can use machines, free weights, or any combination of the two.

A classic circuit strength training program is made up of 10 to 12 training stations. At each station an athlete performs the exercise at 40% to 60% of his or her personal best for 30 to 60 seconds (usually one set of 10–15 repetitions). Between the stations the athlete takes a 30- to 60-second rest. As you will see in this chapter, classic circuit strength training has many variations.

ADVANTAGES

Circuit strength training is used primarily for training beginning athletes; when space, time, and equipment are limited; and in sports that require muscular endurance. It is probably best suited to train athletes involved in muscular endurance sports; these athletes can benefit from the many repetitions, little rest, and submaximum weights used. It can also provide a good in-season maintenance program for many sports.

Young or beginning athletes should start with simple exercises and easy routines to get the body used to strength training. At this level, a workout should be for general fitness and should seem almost like a game, with little emphasis put on lifting heavy weights. Circuit strength training fits this description and gives the athlete muscular strength, muscular endurance, flexibility, and some cardiovascular conditioning.

Classic circuit strength training is a time-saver. Many athletes can train simultaneously with each receiving a good workout in a short time. Because the athlete does only one or two sets per exercise and the rest period between exercises is minimal, the workout can be completed in 30 to 40 minutes.

It is also economical. You can use basic equipment in classic circuit strength training and still get results.

DISADVANTAGES

Classic circuit strength training is not designed for use in programs that require strength/power gains or that have ample time, space, and equipment. Conventional strength training uses more weight, fewer repetitions, and more sets and provides more rest than classic circuit strength training. As a result the two methods give entirely different results. You can set up conventional strength/power training programs in a circuit fashion, but the exercises will be more complex.

In classic circuit strength training each athlete works at 40% to 60% of his or her personal best. Because athletes do so many reps with so little rest time, the intensity is not high enough for optimal strength gains.

Classic circuit strength training does not allow the muscles enough time to recuperate so they can handle heavier weight. For an athlete to develop the ability to handle more weight, muscles need more rest between sets and between exercises.

Though strength increases do occur, they occur much more slowly than in traditional weight training programs. It is also harder to gain muscle bulk and size through circuit strength training.

SETTING UP THE WORKOUT

In classic circuit strength training, athletes usually work out three times a week and should train the whole body at each workout. There must be enough exercises (stations) to train all muscle groups so the total body is strengthened, no matter what sport the athletes are training for. As in other strength training programs, certain areas of the body can be emphasized in addition to the total-body workout.

Exercise Selection

You should select a variety of exercises for classic circuit strength training. Multijoint exercises are especially important because they work many muscles at once. A lot of single-joint exercises will not help the athlete as much as a good variety of multijoint exercises such as the squat, the bench press, and leg presses along with some single-joint exercises.

Also include some exercises that are specific to the sport to improve the athlete's strength in particular areas. For example, wrestlers may emphasize upper-body pulling exercises whereas football players need upper-body pushing exercises. Evaluate the different exercises and the sport, and choose the right combination to do the job. Refer to the section on specificity in chapter 6 (page 51).

Preferably, athletes should first perform the more stressful exercises that train the large muscle groups (e.g., squat, bench) followed by the less stressful ones (the auxiliary exercises). This setup, however, will be affected by the number of athletes training and the number of pieces of equipment you have available.

The recommended number of exercise stations is 10, but you can have as many as 16 depending on how much time and equipment you have. If you include several multijoint exercises, then you need fewer exercises because these train several muscle groups simultaneously. If most of the exercises are single joint or auxiliary ones, then you need more of them.

Because the athletes move from one station to another with minimal rest periods, arrange the stations close together. If your athletes are doing a total-body workout in one day, you should alternate the stations between upper-body and lower-body exercises as much as possible so the different body parts will have a chance to recover before they are trained again. For example, if the athlete moves from the bench press to the leg press to abdominal exercises, each body part has a chance to recover before it is exercised again.

When training athletes in a split routine, alternate between pushing and pulling exercises—for example, the bench press (pushing) followed by lat pulls (pulling), then another pushing exercise. Allow between 30 and 90 seconds of rest between stations. The better trained the athlete, the less rest he or she needs. Also, for greater gains in muscular endurance, the athlete should take shorter rest periods between exercises.

Flow for Circuit Strength Training

Typically athletes proceed through the circuit doing one set of each exercise. If time permits they start the circuit again, doing another set per exercise. For variety, each day start athletes at a different station. For example, say you have 12 stations and 50 athletes to train. Divide the group into 12 smaller groups and have each group start at one of the stations, then rotate (see Figure 7.1).

The Overload Principle and Classic Circuit Training

As in any strength training program, you must use the overload principle when setting up workouts. The athlete's work load must be in-

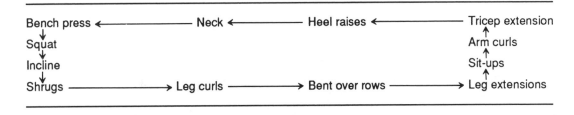

Figure 7.1 Sample flow for a classic circuit strength training routine.

creased for strength gains to occur. There are several ways to increase the work load or make circuit strength training more difficult.

Increase Weight

The most effective way to increase the work load is to increase the weight at each station. If one week the athlete uses 100 pounds and the next week the weight is increased to 110 pounds, he or she is using the overload principle. Be sure the athletes can do the weight you choose in the time available and for the number of repetitions you have specified. For example, if you allow 30 seconds for each exercise and you want the athlete to do 10 reps of that exercise, be sure that he or she can do 10 reps of that weight in the 30 seconds allotted.

Some coaches make the mistake of having each athlete work with preloaded bars or stacks with the same weight for everyone. Many athletes find the weight inadequate for them (too light or too heavy). For best results take the time to get the weights changed to meet each person's needs.

Add Stations

You can add more stations. More work will help the athlete gain in strength. For example, increase an 8-station circuit to 10.

Increase Circuits

Increase the number of circuits. For example, an athlete doing two sets of the exercises (going through the circuit twice) can increase this to three sets; again, the overload principle is being followed.

Increase Reps

Increase the number of repetitions for each set, which also increases the work load. For example, early in the cycle the athlete might do 10 reps of each exercise, and later 12 reps using the same amount of weight. This is for muscle endurance sports.

Decrease Rest

Decrease the rest period between stations. Doing more work in less time is an application of the overload principle. The usual amount of weight used is 40% to 50% of the athlete's 1RM, with sets of 10 to 15 reps. Some very well-trained athletes may be able to do as much as 70% of their 1RM for sets of 10 to 15 reps. Early in the cycle the intensity is 40% to 50% of maximum and is gradually increased each week to end as high as possible, usually 60% to 70% of maximum.

The weight usually remains the same for each set of an exercise (even if the circuit is repeated), but varies from one exercise to another. In some instances the weight is increased from one circuit to the next.

Table 7.1 shows how to increase the intensity from one circuit to the next if the athlete is performing two or three circuits each training day. Usually the first circuit is the lightest, and the weight for each exercise is increased in each subsequent circuit.

ROUTINE VARIATIONS

There are many variations to the traditional circuit strength training routine explained earlier. Variations make the workouts more interesting because your athletes do not have to face the same format day after day. Depending on the sport and the resources available to you, you might find that one of these variations best suits your needs.

The One Set

Athlete A does one set of the required repetitions, then athlete B (partner) does one set.

Table 7.1
Sample of Changes in Intensity With More Than One Circuit the Same Day

Workout	Circuit 1	Circuit 2	Circuit 3
Week 1			
1	40%	40%	45%
2	40%	45%	45%
Week 2			
3	40%	45%	47%
4	40%	45%	50%
Week 3			
5	45%	50%	60%
6	45%	50%	60%
Week 4			
7	45%	55%	65%
8	50%	60%	65%
Week 5			
9	50%	60%	70%
10	50%	60%	70%

They take about a 20- to 30-second rest, move on to the next station, and repeat the alternation. They can repeat the circuit if desired.

The Two Continuous Sets

Athlete A does one set, takes a 10-second rest, and then does the next set. The weight on the second set can be the same or heavier depending on the number of reps performed.

Then athlete B does the same. They then move on to the next exercise. Usually only one circuit is performed.

The Alternate Set

Athlete A does one set, followed by athlete B. Athlete A then does another set, again followed by athlete B. They then move on to the next exercise. The time available will determine how many sets the athletes do at each station. Usually only one circuit is performed.

One Set to Failure

Athlete A does as many repetitions as possible to the point where he or she cannot do any more. Athlete B then does as many as possible until he or she cannot do any more. Then they move on to the next station and work at that exercise all-out. Usually only one circuit is performed.

Timed

Each athlete is ready at his or her station. A whistle is blown and the athlete performs as many reps as possible in a designated amount of time (usually 20–30 seconds). The whistle is blown again; the athlete stops and then moves to another station. This usually takes 20 to 30 seconds; then the whistle is blown again to start the next exercise.

Designing Your Own Program

The right strength training program can make the difference between a winning and a losing season. A winning program is well organized and planned to the last detail. It maps the exact exercises, sets, and reps with the correct intensity and proper amount of rest.

Every team is different. Each has its own set of limitations and requires a program that will work within them. Modeling a program after that of a particular college, professional, or international team is unrealistic. In considering a program for your team ask yourself, "Is it realistic? Does it suit the needs of my athletes?" For example, a muscle magazine may show a power lifter who improves in the bench press by dedicating 2 to 3 hours a day, 4 or 5 days a week to strength training, but the average athlete does not have that kind of time available. Most athletes must also concentrate on schoolwork, sport practice, conditioning, and speed development. They may not be mature enough (physically or psychologically) to handle the sophisticated program of a professional or elite athlete.

BEFORE DESIGNING THE PROGRAM

The following guidelines will help you recognize limitations that can affect your strength training program.

Needs

What are the needs of your athletes? How old are they? Do you want them to gain bulk or muscle endurance? You must evaluate the particular team characteristics.

Time

How much time do your athletes have to train? How many workouts can they perform during the week? Be sure to consider schedule changes, school breaks, and holidays throughout the school year.

Space

How large are your facilities? How many athletes can train at the same time? Are you able to accommodate the entire team at one time, or must you split it into groups?

Equipment

Is a variety of equipment available or only a few pieces? How many of each piece? What exercises can be performed? The equipment you have will dictate what you can do.

Supervision

How many coaches will be in the weight room training the athletes? There should be enough qualified coaches supervising at all times to help the athletes with technique and motivation and to ensure safety.

Knowledge

Can you demonstrate and instruct the athletes in the exercises? If you cannot teach a particular exercise, do not incorporate it into the workout. Otherwise, athletes may do the exercise incorrectly, which poses safety hazards and does not give the results you are looking for.

After you have considered each of the preceding points, move on to designing your program.

STEP 1: ENDURANCE OR STRENGTH/POWER?

Programs can be designed to deliver distinctly different results—muscular strength/power or muscular endurance. Most sports require muscular strength and power (I refer to these as strength/power sports); few require muscular endurance or muscular strength exclusively. If your athletes are going to be standing still in their sport (as in power lifting) then muscular strength is the only thing they need. But because most sports like football, track and field, baseball, volleyball, and basketball require athletes to move quickly with maximum force, players need strength/power. Strength/power gains enable them to be very explosive in the execution of their skills.

If you are not sure whether your athletes need muscular endurance or strength/power, review the following explanations.

Muscular Endurance

Muscular endurance is the ability of the muscle to perform work by continuing to raise and lower a submaximum load. The number of times the muscle contracts against a resistance and the amount of resistance itself must be increased to increase the athlete's muscular endurance. Sports such as wrestling, cross-country running, swimming (long-distance), and most racket sports require muscular endurance. The energy demand of such sports requires the athlete to apply continuous submaximal force.

For athletes to improve their muscular endurance, they must apply the progressive overload principle. Prolonged repetitions of "underloaded" muscle have little effect. The weight must be heavy enough to provide sufficient stimulation. For example, 100 pounds for 15 reps is more beneficial than 70 pounds for 25 reps. Try to increase the load (weight) while maintaining the repetitions between 10 and 15.

In muscular endurance training athletes will also gain strength to a certain extent due to the moderate stress placed on the central nervous system and the development of aerobic energy sources.

Muscular Power

Muscular power is the muscle's ability to release muscular force quickly and explosively. Power is the result of strength and speed and is the most obvious characteristic of a successful athlete. Power can change if the strength or speed components are altered. As the athlete gets stronger he or she is able to generate more power, and as limb speed improves (arms, legs, hips, etc.) the power output increases. For example, an athlete who gains in size and strength while keeping speed the same has gained power because he or she is now bigger and stronger and still moves at the same speed as when he or she was smaller and weaker. Sports like track and field, football, and baseball require energy for short, all-out contractions.

Studies have shown that Olympic-style lifts (power cleans, snatches) require the highest power output of any human movement measured to date. In these lifts the athlete must move the weight quickly to complete the lift.

Because of the weight used and the speed of the movement, the athlete generates power. Include these types of lifts—high pulls, power cleans, and power snatches—in workouts along with the basic strength exercises like squats, benches, and inclines for strength/power gains. A power program involves fewer exercises, heavier weight loads, fewer sets, fewer repetitions, and longer recovery intervals than an endurance program.

Muscular Strength

Muscular strength is the force a muscle can exert against a resistance in one maximum effort. An athlete who can lift more weight than another athlete in a single rep (1RM) is stronger even though the second athlete may be able to lift more weight for 10 repetitions (10RM). To make maximum gains in strength an athlete must overload the muscle. When heavy weights are used for an exercise so that the athlete can perform only a few repetitions, strength is increased at the most rapid rate.

Even though you have evaluated that your athletes' sport—for example, football—requires strength/power, you do not want to train the athletes exclusively with strength/power programs all year long. Early in the off-season some muscular endurance training is necessary to give variety to the training and build a strong base before the athletes begin the long, heavy strength/power program leading up to the season. Similarly, a wrestler might want to do a strength/power program early before doing a specific muscular endurance program to prepare for the season. The two complement each other well when they are integrated at specific times.

STEP 2: YEAR SCHEDULE

After you select what kind of strength program to use, divide the year into training cycles—off-season, preseason, in-season, and active rest. Never train your athletes exactly the same year-round. Each training cycle should be unique and designed to provide a very specific result. The duration of the cycle varies depending on the season, the school year schedule, holidays, and so forth. A cycle can last anywhere between 6 and 12 weeks; I do not recommend longer than 12 weeks because staleness and boredom set in. If you have more than 12 weeks available, divide the time into two cycles. Predetermine the training days and the intensity for each cycle. Test athletes at the end of the cycle to see what they have accomplished and to gain information to use in planning the next cycle. A yearly plan for football might look like the program in Table 8.1.

Let's look at the characteristics of each cycle.

Off-Season

During the off-season the athlete concentrates on the physical demands of the sport and places very little emphasis on practicing the sport skill. It is the longest period of preparation, usually starting a few weeks after the season is over and finishing 1 or 2 months before the next season starts. You can divide the off-season into two or three cycles.

In the early part of the off-season the volume (number of sets and reps) should be high and the intensity (load) low to form a base. As the off-season progresses reduce the number of sets and reps but progressively increase the intensity. For endurance strength training in-

Table 8.1
Sample Yearly Plan

Period	Length	Cycle
December	2 to 4 weeks	Active rest
January to March	8 to 10 weeks	Off-season I
March	2 weeks	Active rest
April to June	8 to 10 weeks	Off-season II
June	2 to 3 weeks	Active rest
June to August	8 weeks	Preseason
September to December	12 to 14 weeks	In-season

crease the intensity while keeping the sets and reps fairly constant. During this time use a variety of general and sport-specific strength training exercises. This is more fully explained later in this chapter in the section on sets and reps.

This is also the time to work on any weaknesses or rehabilitate any injuries that have occurred. At the end of this period the athlete should be well developed in the total body and fully recuperated from any previous problems.

If you have several off-season cycles, each should be more intense than the preceding one to bring the athlete's strength to a higher level.

Preseason

Depending on the sport, this cycle can last from 4 to 8 weeks, ending just before the competition season begins. During this cycle your athletes continue strength training but also begin skills training, conditioning, and practices. Emphasize both conditioning and strength training at this time. Your strength workouts should include more sport-specific exercises. If your athletes require strength/power, incorporate more explosive training (power cleans, high pulls). Athletes perform these exercises with low volume (few repetitions) and high intensity. Those athletes who require muscular endurance should increase loads of the exercises while trying to maintain a very high volume of repetitions and sets. At the end of the preseason cycle the athlete should be ready to meet the demands of his or her particular sport.

In-Season

During this period the athletes spend less time on strength development because of the emphasis on practice and competitions. The number of workouts is reduced. Strength training done during this cycle is used to maintain the strength level gained during the off-season and preseason. Regardless of the sport, athletes must continue some form of strength training; otherwise they will experience significant decreases in strength resulting in decreases in physical capacity or performance. The length of the workouts will vary according to the sport, but they should be short and sharp, very specific to the sport with maximum recuperation time between workouts. For strength/power sports, maintain moderately high intensity and low volume. Endurance athletes should main-

tain a high volume and as high an intensity as possible. Strength training should not interfere with practices or performance in the competitions.

Active Rest

This essential phase is misunderstood, and coaches often neglect to use it to its fullest benefit. You cannot expect athletes to do heavy strength training continuously throughout the year then be ready and fresh when the season starts. Athletes need times during the year when they can slow down to give their bodies a chance to recuperate. This does not mean that they do absolutely nothing but that they should train at a very low stress level. Strength/power athletes should use much lighter weights, and endurance athletes fewer sets and reps. The active rest period gives athletes a chance to recover physically and mentally from the previous hard cycle. Notice where the active rest cycles are placed in Table 8.1. You should take advantage of holidays, vacations, and school closings. The athlete can use this time to stay in shape by doing a variety of fun exercises not related to the sport.

STEP 3: CHOOSING TRAINING DAYS

After you break the year down into cycles, look at the cycles one at a time to see which are the best training days during that cycle (Table 8.2). This will depend on many factors, like weight room availability, class schedules, and practice and competition days. These days are likely to change from cycle to cycle.

Ideally, the athletes will have enough time 3 or 4 days a week to strength train. This is especially helpful in the off-season and during the preseason when you want them to make big strength gains. The following explanation may help you determine which days or what kind of routine to choose.

Total-Body Routines

When training the total body the athlete can train with a Monday-Wednesday-Friday or Tuesday-Thursday-Saturday routine, training the upper and lower body on each day (some

Table 8.2
Sample Routines

Sun	Mon	Tues	Wed	Thur	Fri	Sat
Total body—off-season and preseason						
A. Rest	ST	COND	ST	COND	ST	COND
B. Rest	COND	ST	COND	ST	COND	ST
C. Rest	ST	COND	ST	COND	ST	Rest
Total body—in-season						
A. Rest	PRAC/ST	PRAC	PRAC/ST	PRAC	Compete	Rest
B. Rest	PRAC/ST	PRAC	PRAC/ST	PRAC	Rest	Compete
C. Rest	PRAC	Compete	PRAC/ST	PRAC	Compete	PRAC/ST
Split routine—off-season and preseason						
A. Rest	Upper	Lower	Rest	Upper	Lower	Rest
B. Rest	Lower	Upper	Rest	Lower	Upper	Rest
C. Rest	Upper	Lower	Upper	Lower	Rest	Rest
Split routine—in-season						
A. Rest	UP/PRAC	LO/PRAC	UP/PRAC	PRAC	Compete	Rest
B. Rest	LO/PRAC	UP/PRAC	LO/PRAC	UP/PRAC	Rest	Compete
C. Rest	UP/PRAC	Compete	LO/PRAC	PRAC	Compete	UP/PRAC

Note: ST = strength training, COND = conditioning, PRAC = practice, UP/PRAC = upper body and practice, LO/PRAC = lower body and practice.

states prohibit athletes from participating in school activities on Saturdays). During the season this is cut down to two total-body workouts a week.

Advantages

- The athlete goes into the weight room only 2 or 3 times a week. On the other days he or she can concentrate on the other aspects of his or her sport.
- Because the body is trained as a whole, you can easily incorporate total-body exercises such as the power clean or power snatch into the workouts.
- It can be good for the athletes psychologically to train only three times a week and to stay away from the weight room on some days.

Disadvantages

- Total-body routines require longer training sessions.
- You have to be more careful in selecting the exercises and their order and intensity because the same muscles are being trained three times a week.

Split Routine

The athlete trains the upper and lower body on separate days two times a week—Monday and Thursday for the lower body and Tuesday and Friday for the upper body. This combination requires more workouts, but each workout is shorter. Some athletes may want to use this routine five times a week. If so, they should work one body part three times a week and the other twice. A 6-day routine gives each body part three workouts a week but can easily lead to overtraining and burnout. My recommendation for a split routine is four workouts a week to allow for enough rest.

It is not recommended that athletes use bodybuilder-type training; for example, training the chest and biceps on one day and the triceps and back on another. This can lead to overtraining of certain body parts (e.g., the shoulders).

Advantages

- Because the workouts are shorter, this routine may be easier to use in situations when time is limited.

- If you have many athletes to train in a limited space, a split routine could work well for you. While half the group uses the lower-body equipment, the other half does upper-body work. On the next training day reverse the groups. This allows a large number of athletes to train at the same time, and you make maximum use of the equipment.

Disadvantages

- Even though the athlete is training different body parts on different days, the stress from strength training can accumulate over time.
- Athletes have to do conditioning on the same days as strength training.

Multiple Daily Workouts

We often read that bodybuilders and Olympic lifters train several times during the day, doing workouts in the morning, in the afternoon, and at night. Obviously, this is not applicable to student athletes. Most school programs do not have the time available for this, although some call for a strength training workout in the morning and practice in the afternoon. Olympians and professional athletes are devoted entirely to their sport. Their workouts are often very short, are limited to one or two exercises, and are not full-fledged workouts as some might believe. Because of the many responsibilities student athletes have, they should not attempt to copy this kind of training.

STEP 4: CHOOSING EXERCISES

When choosing strength exercises, keep these four basic points in mind: (a) the maturity of the athletes, (b) an athlete's total-body strength, (c) sport specificity, and (d) antagonistic muscles.

Maturity of the Athletes

You must judge your athletes' maturity and the training level they have achieved. Very young and inexperienced athletes should stay with simple exercises. More mature athletes can do more complex exercises (see Table 8.3).

Table 8.3
Sample Exercises Based on Maturity

Young/inexperienced	Experienced
Total-body exercises	
High pulls	Power cleans
Lower-body exercises	
Leg extensions/leg curls	Squats

Total-Body Strength

For athletic competition the athlete must strengthen the entire body, including all major and minor muscle groups and the stabilizing muscle areas around the joints. To accomplish this you must choose a wide variety of exercises. For example, the athlete should build total leg strength rather than just strong quads. An exercise such as the squat or leg press develops all the major muscles as well as the smaller muscles involved in hip and knee extension. Just doing leg extensions and leg curls does not accomplish this.

Sport Specificity

You should have a basic knowledge of the various anatomical movements used in the sport. Look at how the athlete's body moves in the sport; identify the muscles involved in those movements as well as the predominant muscle groups and at what angle they are working. Select exercises that will strengthen those muscle groups (see Table 8.4).

Table 8.4
Choosing Exercises for Sport Specificity

Type of movement	Muscles used	Exercises
Wrestler Pulling	Biceps and lats	Lat pulldowns Bent-over rows Power cleans Arm curls
Shot-putter Pushing	Triceps and chest	Bench press Incline press Tricep extensions

Antagonistic Muscles

Along with sport-specific exercises, the athlete should do exercises that work the antagonistic (opposite side) muscle groups to develop total-body strength. Body strength should be well balanced.

As you can see in Table 8.5, both athletes will be doing the same exercises, but some exercises are emphasized more than others because they are more specific to the particular sport.

Table 8.5
Choosing Exercises for Antagonistic Training

Type of movement	Sport specific exercises	Antagonistic exercises
Wrestler Pulling	Lat pulldowns Bent-over rolls Power cleans Arm curls	Bench press Incline press Tricep pushdowns
Shot-putter Pushing	Bench press Incline press Tricep extensions	Lat pulldowns Bent-over rolls Power cleans Arm curls

Multijoint Versus Single-Joint Exercises

Strength training exercises can be categorized as either single-joint or multijoint. Usually multijoint exercises are referred to as core exercises and single-joint exercises as auxiliary exercises. Single-joint exercises move only one joint of the body, which contracts one or very few muscles. A good example is the arm curl—the joint is the elbow and the muscle contracted is the bicep. Multijoint exercises move several body joints and muscles. For example, the bench press moves the shoulder and elbow, and the power clean involves the knee, hip, shoulder, and elbow. The more joints that move in a single exercise, the more muscles are worked.

Because multijoint exercises work many muscle groups at the same time, they are the best choice for athletes. A good strength training program includes a combination of multi- and single-joint exercises.

Advantages of Multijoint Exercises

- They are best for strength, power, and size gains (because they train more muscles).
- Many muscle groups working together facilitate the sequential action the athletes perform on the field. For example, the movement of the squat is very similar to that of jumping.
- Because many muscles work at the same time, those muscles are well balanced in strength. Training muscles individually produces a higher chance for imbalance.
- Training the same muscles individually takes a great deal more time. Multijoint exercises reduce workout time; therefore you can train more athletes in less time.
- Multijoint exercises are very popular with athletes and are motivating because athletes can see quicker results.

Disadvantages of Multijoint Exercises

- Multijoint exercises require more coaching and supervision.
- Some multijoint exercises should not be performed by young or inexperienced athletes.

Advantages of Single-Joint Exercises

- You can use single-joint exercises to isolate a particular muscle and give it special attention.
- An injured athlete may not be able to do multijoint exercises and may have to resort to a series of single-joint exercises that isolate the healthy areas. For example, an ankle injury prevents an athlete from doing squats. But he or she can do leg curls, leg extensions, and hip and lower-back exercises to keep those areas strong while giving the injured ankle time to recuperate.

Disadvantages of Single-Joint Exercises

- It takes much longer to isolate each body part than to do multijoint exercises.
- Isolating muscle groups requires a lot of different pieces of equipment.
- An athlete performing single-joint exercises exclusively might ignore the use of stabilizing muscles. Leg extensions and leg curls do not strengthen the knee and hip stabilizing muscles as well as squats or leg presses do.

Bilateral Versus Unilateral Exercises

Most exercises require the use of both arms or both legs working simultaneously (bilaterally). Some exercises require the arms or legs to move one at a time (unilaterally). For example, incline dumbbell presses can be done using first one arm, then the other. For lower-body development, the athlete can do walking lunges or step-ups, exercising one leg at a time.

In bilateral exercises if one side is stronger than the other, the dominant side does more work than the weak side. This is apparent when the athlete can do well in squats (a bilateral exercise) but not in lunges (a unilateral exercise). Lunges, because they work one side at a time, reveal whether or not one leg is weaker than the other. Unilateral exercises not only balance the athlete's strength level but add more joint stability as well. It is not always a lack of strength that prevents an athlete from doing well in unilateral exercises. He or she may simply not have good joint stability in those areas. Lower-body unilateral exercises can be especially helpful in sports that require running or jumping.

Auxiliary Exercises

As I stated earlier, along with the core exercises the athlete should perform a few auxiliary exercises. These are usually used to emphasize a particular area that did not get much work from the core exercises done that day. For example, an athlete who does benches and inclines in the workout can do some arm curls in the auxiliary exercises to work the biceps in an isolated fashion.

You can also help an athlete correct a weakness by assigning auxiliary exercises that zero in on a specific area. For example, an athlete

with weak hamstrings can do leg curls along with squats for extra work in the hamstring area.

Lack of time usually keeps auxiliary work minimal. Therefore it is very important that you select the proper exercises. Certain auxiliary exercises benefit some sports more than others. For example, neck exercises are a must for football and wrestling but not as important for track-and-field athletes.

Recommended Exercises

Some exercises are better than others. Table 8.6 lists the most productive exercises and the areas they strengthen.

STEP 5: ORDER OF EXERCISES

The order in which the athlete performs the exercises is vital to his or her getting the most out of each workout. Apply the "priority training" concept as you prescribe workouts. Priority training means first doing the exercises that logically should be done first and that are most important at the time. Following are six suggestions for deciding the priority of an exercise. You do not have to use all these suggestions at the same time. Choose the ones that suit your particular needs and circumstances.

Complex, Multijoint Exercises First

Athletes should do the most important, most stressful exercises first, follow with less stressful exercises, and leave the auxiliary work for last (Table 8.7). Exercises that work many muscle groups and require a lot of mental concentration (e.g., the power clean) should be performed when the athlete is fresh. Lifts that

Table 8.6
Recommended Exercises

Total body	Upper body	Lower body	Midsection
High pulls	Bench presses	Squats	Hyperextensions
Power cleans	Behind-neck presses	Leg presses	Oblique rotations
Power snatches	Bent-over rows	Lunges	Sit-ups
	Dumbbell presses	Dead lifts	
	Incline presses		

Table 8.7
Sample Exercise Order—Multijoint Exercises First

Order	Exercise
1	Power clean
2	Bench press
3	Dumbbell flies
4	Arm curls

Table 8.9
Sample Exercise Order—Weaker Area First
(Weak Lower Body and Strong Upper Body)

Order	Exercise
1	Squats
2	Lunges
3	Bench press

work small muscle groups and require little concentration (e.g., arm curls) should be performed later as the athlete fatigues.

If auxiliary work is done first, the athlete breaks the balance of the workout. For example, an athlete who does dumbbell flies, training the chest first, and then does the bench press is able to do only as much weight in the bench press as the tired chest muscles will allow. The tricep and shoulder muscles do not get a good workout because they were not pre-exhausted like the chest was.

Higher Intensity First

Always have athletes do the higher intensity exercises first, especially when two exercises work the same muscles (e.g., the bench press and the incline; see Table 8.8). If an athlete does two exercises that train the same area on the same day at different intensities, he or she must do the higher intensity one first while still fresh.

Table 8.8
Sample Exercise Order—Higher Intensity
Exercises First

Exercise	Intensity level
1. Power clean	High
2. Bench press	High
3. Squats	Medium
4. Incline	Medium

Weakest Areas First

Another point of priority training is training the weakest areas first (Table 8.9). For example, an athlete who has a weak lower body and a strong

upper body should do the lower-body exercises first.

Working the weak area first when the athlete is rested results in bigger gains, therefore balancing that weak area over a period of time.

Rotating Emphasis Areas

Priority training can vary from one workout to another. In one workout you may want to place more emphasis on the lower body by having the athlete do those exercises first. In another workout you may want to emphasize the upper body by having the athlete do those exercises first.

Priority training can also be done by exercise. One day the athlete does the squats first, then the bench press, then lunges. Another day lunges are done first, followed by the bench press and the squats (Table 8.10). By rotating the exercises you give them all the same priority. If you always start with the same exercise, that one will improve more rapidly than the others. Rotation assures that all areas get equal emphasis.

Table 8.10
Priority Training by Exercise

Day 1	Day 2
1. Squats	1. Lunges
2. Bench press	2. Bench press
3. Lunges	3. Squats

Push-Pull System

This concept is especially useful in a split routine. If a series of exercises trains the same area, the athlete should not do two exercises back-to-back that work the same muscles (Table 8.11). Alternate pushing and pulling exercises during the workout.

Table 8.11
The Push-Pull Order of Exercises

Upper body	Lower body
1. Bench press (push)	1. Leg press (push)
2. Lat pulldowns (pull)	2. Leg curls (pull)
3. Dumbbell press (push)	3. Leg extensions (push)
4. Arm curls (pull)	

Upper- and Lower-Body Exercises

When the athlete's total body is trained in one day, alternate upper- and lower-body exercises for maximum strength gains (Table 8.12). This gives the muscles time to recuperate before they are trained again. It also enables the athlete to use heavier weights in the exercises. Of course, the athlete should do the more complex and strenuous exercises first, followed by the least complex ones.

Table 8.12
Sample Exercise Order—Upper Body/Lower Body

Exercise
Bench press
Squats
Incline
Lunges
Arm curls
Toe raises

A Sample Week

Let's look at how to choose exercises and in what order they should be performed over a whole week.

As you can see in Table 8.13 a great variety of exercises leads to a well-balanced workout for the week. On Monday the athlete starts with the power clean, which is a power exercise, followed by the bench press and the squat for strength. Then the athlete does lat pulldowns

Table 8.13
Sample of Order of Total-Body Exercises for 1 Week

Monday	Wednesday	Friday
Power clean	Incline	Dead lifts
Bench press	Lunges	Behind-neck press
Back squats	Dumbbell flies	Leg press
Lat pulldown	Leg extensions	Bent-over rows
Tricep extensions	Back raises	Arm curls
Leg curls	Arm curls	Obliques
Sit-ups	Neck exercise	Calf raises

followed by auxiliary work with tricep extensions, leg curls, and sit-ups.

On Wednesday, the athlete emphasizes first the upper body by training the shoulders, then the lower body, then the chest. The auxiliary exercises follow in the same alternating pattern.

Friday the emphasis is placed on the lower body in the dead lift, followed by shoulder exercises, more lower-body work, the lats, and the auxiliary exercises.

STEP 6: REPETITIONS AND SETS

Repetitions are the number of times the athlete does an exercise without resting during one set. An athlete who does 10 push-ups has done 10 repetitions. If this same athlete lifts 200 pounds in the bench twice, he or she is doing two repetitions with 200 pounds. Repetitions are often abbreviated as reps.

A set is the completion of one exercise activity or a number of repetitions performed consecutively without rest. An athlete who lifts 200 pounds in the bench for six reps, takes a short rest, and then does another six reps has done two sets of six reps.

When describing workouts, instead of writing three sets of six reps, we write 3×6. The first number always represents the number of sets and the second, the number of reps.

No single combination of sets and reps yields optimal strength gains in core exercises. What matters most is that as the sets progress the reps are decreased so the athlete can handle more weight (Table 8.14). The number of sets you assign an athlete will vary with the amount of time available and the athlete's work load for that particular time of the year.

Table 8.14
**Sample Muscular Strength Routines
(Sets × Repetitions)**

1. 1 × 8, 2 × 5, 2 × 3
2. 1 × 8, 3 × 5
3. 1 × 8, 1 × 5, 1 × 4, 1 × 3, 1 × 2, 1 × 1

To develop muscular strength/power the athlete should do three to eight repetitions.

For muscular endurance the athlete should do sets of 10 to 15 reps when performing core exercises. Because of the high number of reps, the athlete usually does three or four sets for each core exercise (Table 8.15). Table 8.16 shows some possibilities for set and rep combinations. Again, there is no single best combination.

Table 8.15
**Sample Muscular Endurance Routines
(Sets × Repetitions)**

1. 4 × 10
2. 3 × 15
3. 1 × 10, 1 × 12, 1 × 15

Table 8.16
Sample Sets and Repetitions

Repetitions	Total sets
Core exercises—strength	
8-5-5-3-3	= 5
8-6-5-4-3-2-1	= 7
10-8-5-5-5-5-5	= 7
10-8-5-5-3-3	= 6
10-5-3-5-5	= 5
Core exercises—endurance	
10-10-10-10	= 4
15-15-15	= 3
15-15-12-10	= 4
10-10-10-15	= 4
12-12-12-12	= 4
Auxiliary exercises	
10-10-10	= 3
10-10	= 2
10-8-8	= 3
10-8-6	= 3
10-8	= 2

At the start of a cycle, strength/power athletes perform several sets and reps. As the cycle progresses they perform the same amount of sets but fewer reps to accommodate more weight (Table 8.17). A foundation has to be set before the athlete handles heavy weights.

Table 8.17
**Sample 6-Week Cycle of Bench Press
for a Strength/Power Athlete**

Week	Sets
1	1 × 10, 1 × 8, 4 × 6
2	1 × 10, 1 × 8, 4 × 6
3	1 × 10, 5 × 5
4	1 × 10, 5 × 5
5	1 × 10, 2 × 5, 3 × 3
6	1 × 10, 1 × 8, 1 × 5, 1 × 3, 1 × 1, 1 × 1

The athlete who needs to develop more muscular endurance starts the cycle with several sets and many reps (Table 8.18) and maintains a high number of reps as the season progresses while the weight is increased. Because the reps stay high the athlete is not able to lift as much weight as the person training for strength/power.

Table 8.18
**Sample 6-Week Cycle of Bench Press
for an Endurance Athlete**

Week	Sets
1	4 × 15
2	4 × 15
3	4 × 12
4	4 × 12
5	4 × 10
6	4 × 10

The preceding examples apply to the core exercises but not the auxiliary exercises. Because the auxiliary exercises usually train one muscle group, the athlete performs them at high reps with few sets, as for muscular endurance. These exercises are performed in three or four sets of 8 to 12 reps. If time is limited you can reduce this to one or two sets for each exercise.

STEP 7: HOW MUCH WEIGHT?

Before you start this section, you must understand that all weights are based on percentages of the maximum the athlete can do (personal best) for a single repetition, or 1RM. Using percentages assures that each athlete is working at his or her own level, no matter how strong he or she is. The following percentages represent the last set for each exercise. How much weight should be used in the other sets is explained in step 8 of this chapter.

Starting Weights

Starting weights depend on when the last cycle ended and the athlete's physical condition at the beginning of the current cycle. An athlete who does two cycles close together with only a week of rest between them will be able to start the next cycle at up to 65% to 75% of his or her personal best (1RM). If, however, there are several weeks of active rest, the athlete is not in as good a shape and should begin with a lower intensity (50% to 65% of his or her personal best).

The starting weight also depends on how many sets and reps the athlete starts with. If he or she starts with sets of many repetitions (10–15 reps) the starting intensity should be lower. The higher the number of repetitions, the lower the intensity. On the other hand, an athlete who trains heavy early in the cycle should use fewer sets and reps to accommodate the heavier weights (Table 8.19).

Table 8.19
Guide for Starting Intensities
at the Beginning of a Cycle

Low repetitions (5 to 8)	High repetitions (10 to 15)
In shape 65% to 75%	In shape 50% to 60%
Not in shape 50% to 65%	Not in shape 40% to 50%

Intensity Week by Week

The next step is breaking down the cycle into different weeks. Use a percentage of the athlete's projected new RM, which is the goal you would like the athlete to achieve at the end of the cycle, as a guide in determining how much weight the athlete should use each week. For example, say you have an athlete who is going to bench press heavy once a week for an 8-week cycle. The cycle follows a long active rest period, so the athlete starts the first week doing sets with high reps at about 60% of his or her 1RM (Table 8.20). This intensity may seem low, but early in the cycle it may be all the athlete can handle. As the weeks go by, you can increase the intensity as the athlete gets stronger and as the number of reps are decreased. The athlete should achieve the new RM in the last weeks of the cycle. Step 8 in this chapter explains how much weight to use in the sets that lead up to the last heavy set.

At the end of the cycle you should see a new personal best with an improvement of between 5% and 20% depending on the athlete's experience and maturity level and the length of the cycle. The longer the cycle, the greater the athlete's chance of improvement over the previous cycle. Usually less experienced athletes show greater improvement than advanced athletes. Remember to consider the length of the training cycle and the athlete's maturity when you project his or her new 1RM at the end of the cycle.

This is a very rough guideline of a planned cycle. You may have to make adjustments during the cycle. Keep an eye on the athlete's weekly progress and make any small changes that are necessary. As you gain experience you will become more adept at projecting results.

Intensity Within the Week

There is evidence that an athlete makes more progress if he or she does not use maximum weight each time the exercise is done. An athlete who does the same lift twice during the week should perform it one day at a heavy intensity and the other at a lighter intensity.

Intensity is relevant to the point in the cycle. The athlete may have a 400-pound 1RM; obviously he or she cannot handle that amount of weight at the beginning of the cycle. The first workout may be with 250 pounds (60%) for 10 reps. If that is all the athlete can handle at that point, it is an all-out effort, or heavy workout. If the athlete does that same exercise again during the week, he or she should do it at a lighter intensity. For example, change the 250 pounds to 225 pounds for 10 reps. The next week you may be able to increase the weight to 280 pounds (65%) for 10 reps for the heavy workout and 240 pounds for the lighter workout. The lighter intensity is 5% to 15% lower than the heavy intensity of that week. A heavy workout does not necessarily mean that an athlete does singles with a maximum weight. A set of 10 reps with as much weight as the athlete can handle is considered a heavy workout, because the athlete is going all out.

For example, say an athlete will be doing the bench press two times a week. Using the same example shown in Table 8.20, you can see that for a light workout the athlete performs the same combination of sets and reps but at a lower intensity (Table 8.21).

STEP 8: COMBINING EXERCISES, SETS, REPS, AND INTENSITY

Now that you have chosen the exercises the athlete should do during the cycle and determined the intensity at which you would like him or her to start, it is time to incorporate these into the actual workout. To simplify your job and the athlete's, refer to the four different sample charts described in the next paragraphs. Post complete versions of them at each training station.

The first sample chart (Table 8.22) explains the workout for the day—which exercises the athletes are to do, how many sets and reps, and

Table 8.20
8 Weeks of the Bench Press

Weeks	Sets × Reps	Intensity
1	3 × 10	60%
2	4 × 10	65%
3	1 × 8, 5 × 5	70%
4	1 × 8, 5 × 5	75%
5	1 × 8, 5 × 5	80%
6	1 × 8, 2 × 5, 3 × 3	85%
7	1 × 8, 1 × 5, 2 × 3, 1 × 2	90%
8	1 × 8, 1 × 5, 1 × 3, 1 × 2, 1 × 1	100%

Note: % represents weight handled on the last set.

Table 8.21
Intensity Within the Week

Weeks	Sets × Reps	Heavy	Light
1	3 × 10	60%	55%
2	4 × 10	65%	60%
3	1 × 8, 5 × 5	70%	65%
4	1 × 8, 5 × 5	75%	70%
5	1 × 8, 5 × 5	80%	75%
6	1 × 8, 2 × 5, 3 × 3	85%	75%
7	1 × 8, 1 × 5, 2 × 3, 1 × 2	90%	80%
8	1 × 8, 1 × 5, 1 × 3, 1 × 2, 1 × 1	100%	85%

at what intensity. Prepare this chart daily or weekly. The athlete sees the workout for the day and the order of rotations.

On the second sample (Table 8.23) the new projected personal best (RM) of each member of the team is listed by core exercise. Test athletes at the end of every cycle and set a new RM for each athlete for each core exercise. Update the chart by writing down each athlete's new RMs after each test.

The third sample chart (Table 8.24) gives the percentages for each weight listed (see Appendix A for the full chart). This is a standard chart and will not change.

The fourth sample chart (Table 8.25) is a weight progression chart (see Appendix B for the full chart). This also is a standard chart. You may use the sample chart or make one of your own.

How to Use the Charts

By using the sample workout in Table 8.22 and the sample personal bests in Table 8.23, you can follow the process step-by-step to learn how to use the charts. These charts will make it easier for you to write workouts for your athletes.

Using Pat and Chris as subjects, let's look at a couple of ways to use the charts. Pat's workout for day 1 calls for the power clean for 1×8, 2×5, 2×3, and 1×1 at 95%. First Pat looks up his personal best in the power clean. The chart shows 270 pounds. Then he looks at the percentage chart (see Table 8.24 for example, and Appendix A for full chart) to find out what 95% of 270 would be.

The chart shows 255 pounds. Now, Pat knows that his last set (single rep) should be done at 255 pounds. To find out how much weight should be used in his other sets he looks at the weight progression chart (Table 8.25).

The chart shows 135-155-185-215-235-255. His power clean workout for the day, therefore, should be 135×8, 155×5, 185×5 (two sets of five reps), 215×3, 235×3 (two sets of three reps), 255×1. Chris's workout for day 1 calls for the bench press at 1×8, 5×5 at 75%. Chris finds his personal best in the bench press—350 pounds. Then he finds 75% of 350 pounds from the percentage chart (Table 8.26).

The chart shows 265 pounds. Chris knows that his last set of five should be done with 265 pounds. To find out how much weight should be used in his other sets he looks at the weight progression chart (Table 8.27).

Table 8.22
Sample Workouts

Day 1			Day 2		
Power clean			Power clean		
1×8, 2×5, 2×3, 1×1		95%	1×8, 2×5, 2×3, 3×3		75%
Bench press			Incline		
1×8, 5×5		75%	1×8, 5×5		75%
Squat			Squat		
1×8, 2×5, 3×3		80%	1×8, 2×5, 3×3		70%
Auxiliary exercises			Auxiliary exercises		

Table 8.23
Projected Personal Best

Name	Bench	Power clean	Squat	Incline
Pat Strong	300	270	430	260
Chris Huge	350	300	570	280
Mary Fitt	100	80	205	80

Table 8.24
Sample From Percentage Chart

Weight	40%	45%	50%	55%	60%	65%	70%	75%	80%	85%	90%	95%
260	105	120	130	145	155	170	180	195	210	220	235	245
270	110	125	135	150	160	175	190	200	215	230	245	**255**
280	110	125	140	155	170	180	195	210	225	240	250	265

Table 8.25
Sample From Weight Progression Chart

Set 1	Set 2	Set 3	Set 4	Set 5	Set 6
135	155	185	210	220	250
135	**155**	**185**	**215**	**235**	**255**
135	155	185	220	240	260

Table 8.26
Sample From Percentage Chart

Weight	40%	45%	50%	55%	60%	65%	70%	75%	80%	85%	90%	95%
340	135	155	170	190	205	220	240	255	270	290	305	325
350	140	160	175	195	210	230	245	**265**	280	300	315	335
360	145	160	190	200	220	230	250	270	290	310	320	340

Table 8.27
Sample From Weight Progression Chart

Set 1	Set 2	Set 3	Set 4	Set 5	Set 6
135	155	185	220	240	260
135	**155**	**185**	**225**	**245**	**265**
135	155	185	230	250	270

The chart shows 135-155-185-225-245-265. His bench workout for the day, therefore, should be 135 × 8, 155 × 5, 185 × 5, 225 × 5, 245 × 5, 265 × 5.

Both athletes apply the same steps to each of their exercises to complete the total workout. If a specific core exercise is to be performed for a total of five sets, use the first five columns in the weight progression chart to find the specific weights the athlete does for each set. If the exercise is to be performed for four sets, use the first four columns in the weight progression chart.

Intensity for Auxiliary Exercises

Follow these steps when entering weights for auxiliary exercises. Use the Auxiliary Exercise Weight Progression Chart in Appendix C.

1. Because auxiliary exercises are at the end of the workout athletes do not need to do many warm-ups for each exercise. As the chart shows, the weights of the three sets are relatively close, progressing for each set. The weight in the last set should be as heavy as the athlete can handle for the amount of repetitions prescribed.

2. Refer to the previous week's workout. If all sets and reps were completed for each auxiliary exercise, the athlete should be able to use a heavier weight.

Example:

Arm curls

Last week	This week
30 × 8	35 × 8
40 × 8	45 × 8
45 × 8	50 × 8

In this example last week's sets were done at 30, 40, and 45 pounds, and all reps were performed as prescribed. This week the athlete can go to the next line on the progression chart.

Set 1	Set 2	Set 3
30	40	45
35	45	50
40	50	55

3. If the athlete did not complete all the sets or reps in the previous workout, have him or her stay with the same progression this week until the athlete can complete them. For example, if in the last set of 45-pound arm curls the athlete could do only six reps, he or she should stay with the same progression until all reps in the last set can be completed. Only then should you increase the weight in the next workout.

4. If the athlete will be doing only two sets for a particular exercise, use the first two numbers from the set column.

Intensity for Down Sets

"Down sets" are done after the heaviest set has been completed. Down sets are for muscle growth. First the athlete does a good progression leading up to the heavy weights, which will result in strength gains. Then, a few down sets will give additional muscle mass for further strength gains. Follow these instructions for entering the weight for down sets.

All down sets are based on an athlete's heaviest set. If after an athlete has completed the heaviest set he or she is supposed to do two down sets, subtract the amount of weight indicated on the workout form from the athlete's heaviest set.

Example:
Bench Press
135 × 8
155 × 5
185 × 5
205 × 5
225 × 5 (75%)
205 × 8 (−20)
205 × 8 (−20)

STEP 9: REST AND RECUPERATION

Rest is as much a part of strength training as the exercises themselves. During rest periods the muscles grow and get stronger. Insufficient rest during the workout or between workouts can impair an athlete's progress toward greater strength.

Rest Between Repetitions

No rest should be taken between repetitions. Some athletes tend to do this, especially in stressful exercises such as power cleans, heavy squats, or benches. But resting between repetitions will not have the same training effect, because these are actually several singles, not a set. Rest is taken only after a set is completed.

Rest Between Sets

The amount of rest necessary between sets depends upon the desired results of the workout. For muscular endurance the athlete needs only 30 to 60 seconds between sets, performing one set after another.

For muscular strength, however, more rest (2 minutes) between sets is needed. If the intensity is very high the athlete may need from 3 to 5 minutes between sets. It takes about 30 seconds for half of the muscles' energy to be restored and up to 3 minutes before nearly all energy is restored. Less than 1 minute of rest between sets does not permit the muscles to restore adequate energy for high intensity (heavy weights) performances.

Taking too much rest (5–10 minutes), on the other hand, will cause the athlete to cool down, which breaks the continuity of the exercise and increases the chance of injury.

Rest Between Exercises

The amount of rest taken between exercises depends on the muscle groups exercised that day and whether the athlete is training for muscular strength or endurance. In a total-body routine, alternating upper- and lower-body exercises within the workout allows one body part to recuperate while the other works. Consequently, the amount of rest needed between exercises is minimal (60 to 90 seconds). For example, after doing bench presses and before doing military presses, an athlete could do leg presses, which allow the athlete's upper body to recuperate for military presses. In a split routine, however, more rest is needed between exercises (2–3 minutes) because all the exercises work one specific area.

For muscular endurance gains the exercises should be done with little rest (30–60 seconds) between them. But for muscular strength gains you need much more rest (2–5 minutes) between exercises.

Rest Between Workouts

The recovery period between workouts is one of the most misunderstood and neglected factors of strength training. Muscles do pump up during the workout, but this is not actual muscle growth, merely the muscles' immediate response to the stress being placed on them. It is during the time between workouts that the muscles restore themselves and get stronger.

When a muscle is stressed beyond its normal capacity, a certain amount of time is necessary for it to recover. If the time between workouts is too short the muscle will become chronically fatigued and will actually decrease in strength. Although some athletes require more recuperation time than others, 48 to 72 hours rest between workouts on the same muscle groups is probably sufficient. This means that no athlete should do more than three total-body workouts a week (e.g., on Monday, Wednesday, and Friday or on Tuesday, Thursday, and Saturday). A split routine may be done four times a week but training sessions on the same muscle area should be separated by at least 48 hours (e.g.,

upper body, Monday and Thursday; lower body, Tuesday and Friday).

Rest Between Training Cycles

At the end of a competitive season or a period of hard training the athlete should slow down. This slow-down is called the active rest period. No one can train hard all year long without resting. Continuous training will lead to overtraining, boredom, and lower strength gains. In order to ensure that the athlete will rest, the year is divided into several strength training cycles of 6 to 12 weeks each. At the end of each training cycle the athlete should take 1 or 2 weeks of active rest before beginning the next cycle. The length of the active rest period depends on the time available to the athlete and the intensity of the previous training period. Take advantage of holidays, vacations, and school closings for active rest periods. This is a time for the athlete to train lightly (fun exercises like arm curls, dips, pull-ups) and recuperate before starting a new training period.

STEP 10: VARIETY FROM CYCLE TO CYCLE

One of the main problems of strength training is simply maintaining the enthusiasm of the trainee so he or she does not drop out of the program. A poorly designed strength program can be boring. If the athlete has to do the same exercises and the same number of sets and reps over and over again, he or she will lose interest. When planning the different cycles, try to introduce variations that will help an athlete stay interested in achieving the goals you have set. Look for new methods of arranging the same variables of duration, load distribution, order of exercises, sets and reps, and rest time. These changes will help keep the athlete motivated and the muscles stimulated for bigger strength gains.

Because the athlete will be involved in two or more off-season cycles, not every off-season cycle should be exactly like the other. They should all lead to the desired result of strength gains, but they should have variety. Change the order or kind of exercises from one cycle to the next, but train the same muscle groups. For example, in one cycle the athlete might use the incline bench press to train the upper body, and on the next cycle the athlete might use incline dumbbells. These two exercises train the same muscle groups, but the variety helps the athlete maintain interest in reaching new goals.

Vary the Sets and Reps

Variety in the sets and reps is also critical in continuing the progress of the athletes and keeping them motivated. Variety in two 8-week off-season cycles might look like Table 8.28. All percentages are based on projected goals.

STRENGTH PROGRAM FOR THE MULTISPORT ATHLETE

Most coaches are aware of the demands placed on athletes who participate in more than one sport (sometimes as many as three) during the school year. These athletes are often the most talented of all, and they should be wary of the amount and type of strength training they do.

It is important that multisport athletes and all coaches involved with them cooperate with each other. In addition to specific training for their sport, multisport athletes must continue overall strength training. Too often, sport coaches forbid their players to strength train during the competition season. This is wrong in itself, but it is especially detrimental to the athlete who will compete in another sport in the next season. Do not let your personal philosophy, however, interfere with these athletes' training and consequently undermine their performance in upcoming sports. Be aware of multisport athletes' special situations, and help to maintain their overall strength training programs.

Maintaining Strength Levels

During the season or multiple seasons, the athlete will not make large gains in strength. Most training is geared toward maintaining strength that was gained in the off-season or preseason. With classes, practices, and games, there is not enough time to make big gains.

There are two basic guidelines when training multisport athletes: (a) athletes must continue strength training regardless of the sport in which they are currently participating, and (b) two workouts minimum per week are necessary to maintain strength, and the athlete should train the upper and lower body in each workout. If the athlete cannot train at least two days a week, the workouts should be done during school holidays, breaks, and game cancellations. In other words, the athlete should add a strength training workout any time it will not interfere with the sport in which he or she is participating.

Table 8.28
Varying the Sets and Reps in Strength Workouts

Cycle 1			Cycle 2		
Week 1	3 × 10	60%	Week 1	3 × 8	65%
Week 2	4 × 10	65%	Week 2	4 × 8	70%
Week 3	2 × 8, 3 × 5	70%	Week 3	1 × 8, 4 × 6	74%
Week 4	2 × 8, 3 × 5	75%	Week 4	1 × 8, 4 × 5	78%
Week 5	2 × 8, 3 × 5	80%	Week 5	1 × 8, 1 × 5, 4 × 4	82%
Week 6	1 × 8, 2 × 5, 3 × 3	85%	Week 6	1 × 8, 1 × 5, 4 × 3	86%
Week 7	1 × 8, 2 × 5, 3 × 3	90%	Week 7	1 × 8, 1 × 5, 4 × 2	92%
Week 8	1 × 8, 1 × 5, 1 × 3, 1 × 2, 1 × 1	100%	Week 8	1 × 8, 1 × 5, 1 × 3, 1 × 2, 1 × 1	100 + %

CHAPTER

9

Testing and Evaluation

Testing and evaluation are positive and constructive elements of strength training; they help show how athletes are progressing and serve as a gauge of your overall program; they provide motivation for athletes and give them a chance to show their stuff. Athletes who are regularly tested and evaluated will work harder and show improvement in performance.

Testing should be well planned and done only for a specific purpose. Do not test just for the sake of testing. Because testing takes time away from training, make sure you are testing at the right time and for the right purpose.

The age and maturity of the athletes will dictate what kind of testing and how often the testing is done. Strength testing for novices should be kept simple and done often to help motivate them. Testing more advanced athletes can involve higher expectations and more difficult exercises but might be done less often. Advanced athletes know training leads to better results, and they are motivated by that.

WHY TEST?

I have found there are various reasons for testing.

Motivation

The most important reason for testing is to give the athletes a chance to give an all-out effort and show the coach and team that they have met their goals. Continuous training without a goal does not motivate. Athletes are motivated when they can show what they can do, compete with others, and get psyched about improving.

Accountability

If the athletes know they will be tested they will take the responsibility to train hard. They know they will have to prove to the coach and teammates that they have done the work and are contributing to the success of the team.

Upgrading of Workouts

In order to train athletes at higher levels you must have up-to-date measurements of their strength. Workouts in the next cycle will take into consideration the new gains in strength. This will enable you to make workouts much more specific to athletes' new strength levels and keep up with the progress of each athlete.

Program Validation

The individual and team test results will help you evaluate your strength training program. You can determine if the program needs changes and what those changes should be. Were correct exercises chosen? Were correct levels of sets and reps established? Was the week-by-week intensity too low or too high? Test results will tell if the right changes were made.

Talent Search

Strength testing can give an indication if an athlete is strong and physically prepared enough to play a particular sport or position. If an athlete has good strength and body weight, for example, he might be a football lineman.

Recognition of Weaknesses

Results from a battery of tests will highlight athletes' weaknesses or muscle imbalances. Recognizing these problems will help you stabilize or strengthen the specific muscle areas before injury occurs. This is especially important to young athletes. Testing gives a more accurate picture of what the athlete is able to do and where improvements should be made.

Proper Peaking

Athletes should be at their peak level at just the right time, not 2 months earlier or later. By testing at the proper time (e.g., before the season starts) you can schedule workouts accordingly to help your athletes excel at the right time of year.

WHEN TO TEST?

Depending on the purpose, testing can be done at any time of the year. But do not go into it blind and without planning. Random testing does not apply to strength training—the athletes must have time to train. The most common testing times are (a) before the start of a cycle (pre-testing) and (b) at the end of a cycle (post-testing).

Pre-testing is used to determine strength levels at the start of a cycle. This is especially important with athletes just entering the program.

Those who are already part of the program do not need to be pre-tested.

Because new athletes are not prepared to lift a lot of weight at the beginning of a new cycle, you must be very careful in administering strength tests at this time. Do not use maximum attempts in pre-testing. Instead, use submaximum testing—the athletes handle less weight with more repetitions, thus decreasing the chance of injury. (See "Which Tests?" in this chapter.) If you still want to see a 1RM, monitor the test very carefully and remember, the athlete was not training hard before the test.

Post-testing is done at the end of a cycle to see if the preset goals have been met. This is the best and most productive time to test. Because it is at the end of a training cycle, heavy weight can be handled, and the athlete is more capable of giving an all-out effort and a true indication of his or her new level of strength.

If you want to administer several tests during the year, remember that testing takes time away from training. Too many tests decrease their effectiveness, so keep them to a minimum. Testing should be done before the season, at the end of preseason training, and, if desired, at the end of the playing season. Volleyball players, for example, should be tested at the end of summer, just before the season starts. Tests from the end of the season will show how much strength was maintained during the season and whether in-season training was productive. Testing should also be done at the end of each cycle during the off-season. These results can be compared to those from the previous cycle and to those from the same time the previous year. These comparisons will show the progress made.

WHICH TESTS?

Depending on the sport and your personal preference there are two different tests you may administer: (a) 1RM test and (b) submaximum test for reps.

1RM Test

In this test the athlete tries to lift as much weight as possible for one repetition. This type of test is a good indication of brute strength. It is usually administered to football players, sprinters, shot-putters, and other athletes that require power. Some exercises to use in this testing are the squat, bench press, incline, behind-the-neck press, power clean, or dead lift. This type of test is not recommended for testing auxiliary exercises such as arm curls or leg extensions.

Submaximum Test for Reps

In this test the athlete uses a submaximum weight (70%–85% of estimated 1RM) and does as many repetitions with that weight as he or she can. To get an estimated 1RM use the chart shown in Table 9.1 and match the workout weight the person has been using with the number of reps he or she has done. Then look to the one-repetition column for an estimated maximum weight. For strength/power sports you should use 80% to 85% of 1RM. For muscular endurance sports such as distance running, wrestling, and rowing, use 70% of 1RM and have the athlete do as many reps as possible. The best exercises to use in this testing can be the same as the ones done for 1RM testing except the Olympic-style lifts (power clean, snatch). If you are testing auxiliary exercises, use 70% of the calculated max and have the athletes do as many repetitions as they can. Refer to Table 9.1 on p. 84.

WHAT TO TEST?

After you have chosen what type of test you will use, keep these points in mind.

- Test the area you have asked the athlete to work on. If you have had the athlete doing squats, do not test in the leg press.
- Test areas that are motivational to the athlete. A good example is the bench press, which athletes love. Even though in certain sports the bench press is not as important as other exercises, you may want to test in the bench press anyway because it motivates the athlete. This does not mean you should test only those exercises the athletes like, but include tests on exercises that are meaningful and motivational to them.
- Because there are so many exercises the athlete will perform and so little time actually to test, not all exercises will be tested on testing day. Some exercises can be evaluated, however, during regular workouts

with what is called "objective testing." If you are not able to test the athlete, for example, in the incline press, you can refer to the weights the athlete used during the last few workouts. Use the personal best conversion chart (Table 9.1) to see what would be his or her new 1RM in the incline press. For example, if in workouts the athlete did 225 pounds for 3 reps, his or her estimated personal best in the incline press would be 240 pounds, as the chart shows.

- Test exercises specific to the sport. Total-body strength is important, but certain sports and positions require athletes to be stronger in one area and possibly more. For example, you may want to test a wrestler's shoulder strength. You should therefore test the wrestler on behind-the-neck presses. The squat gives an indication of leg strength, and the power clean gives an indication of total-body strength.

HOW TO TEST?

Let the athletes know when you are going to test. This gives them time to prepare, physically and mentally. If it is not possible to set aside specific testing days, regular workout days can be used, but again the athletes need to know in advance of the day they will be evaluated. Whatever system you use, make the athletes look forward to test day by making it an important event.

Before you look at the general guidelines of testing, look at a few things that are very important when administering a test.

Is the Test Valid?

Is the test going to give you the information you are really looking for? For example, if you want to see upper-body strength, you should make sure the test will give that information. For information on upper-body strength, a 1RM bench press test is much more valid than a test on how many push-ups an athlete can do.

Is the Test Reliable?

The test must be administered in exactly the same manner for each athlete, from one trial to the next, and from one year to the next. If

Table 9.1
Personal Best Conversion Chart

				Number of repetitions					
10	9	8	7	6	5	4	3	2	1
115	115	120	120	125	130	135	140	145	150
115	120	125	130	135	140	145	150	155	160
125	130	135	140	145	150	155	160	165	170
135	140	145	150	155	160	165	170	175	180
145	150	155	160	165	170	175	180	185	190
155	160	165	170	175	180	185	190	195	200
160	170	175	180	185	190	195	200	205	210
170	180	185	190	195	200	205	210	215	220
175	185	190	195	200	205	210	215	220	230
185	195	200	205	210	215	220	225	230	240
190	200	205	210	215	220	230	235	240	250
200	210	215	220	225	230	240	245	250	260
205	215	220	225	230	235	245	250	260	270
215	220	230	235	240	245	255	260	270	280
225	230	235	240	245	250	260	270	280	290
235	240	245	250	255	260	270	280	290	300
240	250	255	260	265	270	280	290	300	310
245	255	260	265	270	280	290	300	310	320
255	265	270	275	280	290	300	310	320	330
260	270	280	285	290	300	310	320	330	340
270	275	285	290	300	310	320	330	340	350
275	280	290	295	305	310	325	340	350	360
280	285	295	305	315	330	335	345	355	370
290	295	305	315	325	340	345	355	365	380
300	305	310	325	335	350	355	360	375	390
310	315	320	330	345	355	365	375	385	400
315	325	335	345	355	365	375	385	395	410
325	335	345	355	365	375	380	390	405	420
335	345	355	365	375	385	395	405	415	430
345	355	365	375	385	395	405	415	425	440
355	365	375	385	395	405	415	425	435	450
360	370	380	390	400	415	425	435	445	460
365	385	395	405	415	425	425	445	455	470
370	390	405	415	425	435	445	455	465	480
380	400	415	425	435	445	455	465	475	490
385	410	420	430	445	455	465	475	485	500
400	420	430	440	455	465	475	485	495	510
405	425	435	450	460	475	485	495	505	520
410	430	440	455	465	480	490	500	515	530
415	440	450	465	475	490	500	515	525	540
425	450	465	475	490	500	515	525	535	550
435	460	475	485	500	515	525	535	545	560
440	470	480	490	505	525	535	545	555	570
445	475	485	500	510	530	540	555	565	580
455	480	495	510	525	535	550	565	575	590
460	480	500	515	530	545	555	575	585	600

methods change from one administration to another, the test becomes unreliable. Do not change your procedures. Make sure you use the same type of warm-up, the same apparatus, the same technique, and the same testing criteria.

Is the Test Simple and Economical?

Do you have the necessary equipment, personnel, and time to administer the tests? Some complex tests cannot be administered for lack of time and equipment. Be realistic and use only those tests you can administer with what resources you have.

Is the Test Interesting?

Encourage competition to stimulate the athletes to do their best. If the test is boring and undemanding, the athletes will not give it all they have, and the test will not measure optimal performance. Have all athletes and coaches present during testing as a way to make the day more interesting. Have everyone encourage each other and get excited about testing. Testing is the final reward at the end of a training cycle.

GENERAL GUIDELINES FOR TESTING

Consider these basic guidelines for use before and during testing.

- Instruct your athletes to warm up adequately before testing. Warm-ups will prevent injury and let athletes practice the exercise.
- Have your athletes use training aids as they do during normal training sessions. If the athlete never does exercises using training aids (supersuits, wraps, or straps), they should not be used during testing. If the athlete uses a lifting belt during training, then one should also be worn during testing.
- Use the same technique as that used during training. The athlete should not be called

upon to do anything special during testing. Attempts not done correctly do not count, and the athlete should be aware of this before the test. For example, in squats, parallel means parallel; in the bench press, touch and go means touch and go, not bounce.
- Use the same equipment. Differences in equipment will make a difference in results. If you are going to test the bench press with free weights, you cannot test the next time with a machine. Even a different kind of bench press can make a difference. If the athlete normally uses the same apparatus but now has to use a new or different apparatus, the test results can be different.
- Administer tests at the same time of day. Testing early in the morning might result in poorer performance than testing in the afternoon. Be consistent.
- Give the same amount of rest before testing days. If the athlete had a hard running workout before one test day but did not another time, it will make a difference in the results. Adequate recovery time from workouts must be given to get an all-out effort on testing days.
- Do not test the same athlete in several strength tests on the same day. The later tests will not give good indications of strength because the athlete is tired from the previous tests. Distribute the strength tests over several days to give the athlete time to recuperate. For example, if you want to test two upper-body exercises and two lower-body exercises, you might want to split them up into two days. Do one upper and lower exercise one day, allow a day of rest, and do the other upper and lower exercises the third day.
- For the same tests taken in two different training cycles, consider the athletes' outside activities. Activities done outside the weight room during training cycles will make a difference on testing results. Tests from a cycle in which the athlete is just doing strength training will differ from tests done during a cycle in which the athlete was doing strength training and a lot of running. The more activities the athlete does outside the weight room, the lower the strength gains will be.

- Use the same coach as judge. People may have different testing procedures. What one judge may call a good lift another may not. The supervising coach should also see all attempts to ensure accuracy of the numbers and of the technique.
- Allow trials. When doing a 1RM after warm-ups, the athlete should be allowed several trials to reach a certain weight. If the athlete is doing a submaximal test or a muscular endurance test, he or she should do the warm-ups, go straight to the assigned weight, and do as many reps as possible.
- Explain the warm-ups you have chosen for the athlete to reach his or her personal best. The weight progression should not tire the athlete during warm-ups. Most athletes want to do too much weight in the warm-up. Refer to the Weight Progression Chart in Appendix B or C. This chart shows the proper selection of weight for each set.
- Allow retrials at lower weights. An athlete who tries to lift a certain weight but misses should have the opportunity to try again at the same weight or a lighter weight. After all, you are trying to determine the best the athlete can do, not staging a lifting competition. Usually, an athlete can try three or four times at a heavy weight before fatigue sets in. Be sure, if this is the case, the athlete has adequate rest (5 minutes) between trials.
- Be conservative in testing procedures. If you do not know the athlete's strength capabilities, use very light weights to start and increase gradually. When you see a breakdown in technique or excessive strain, stop the test.

ORGANIZATION OF THE TESTING DAY

You need to be well organized and do everything possible to facilitate the athletes' efforts. Therefore, you should follow these guidelines:

- Test small groups at a time. If possible, these groups should be at the same strength levels to make the testing more competitive. As added motivation, the other athletes can watch and encourage the ones testing.

Squad size will determine how many small groups you will have and how long the test will last. Try to get some help and allow plenty of time so as not to rush the athletes.

- If possible, do only one strength test per day. If more than one coach is available, then more than one test can be done during that particular time.
- Have all the paper work ready to record the results. The exact progression should be given to each athlete or posted by the apparatus. The old personal best of each athlete and goals that were set should also be posted.

USING TEST RESULTS

After the testing is completed you need to use the results to help you validate the program and to motivate the athletes. There are several ways you can do this.

Comparing Test Results Against Other Programs

Be very careful when comparing your results with another team or school. Comparing your school to another school is unfair unless you know the exact criteria being used. For example, some coaches have their athletes do only half squats instead of full squats but will say they have a certain number of athletes who can squat over 400 pounds. If you are doing full squats in your program, it might be difficult to get the same number of athletes to do over 400 pounds. Another way that tests from other schools can differ from yours is that they may use different techniques or place emphasis in an area that you do not. What should be important to you is how your athletes are progressing, not how they compare to other programs.

Comparing Test Results Within the Team

In comparing test results within your own team be sure that you are comparing results under similar circumstances. Results will be different at different times of the year because of factors such as practices, conditioning workouts, and length of cycle, among others. See the general guidelines for testing listed previously to find out what other factors affect test results.

Be careful also not to compare players because of the many differences between athletes (age, size, maturity, etc.).

For reliable evaluation of progress use the following.

- Compare results from one off-season cycle to results from another off-season cycle in the same year.
- Compare off-season and preseason results in the same year to see total progress during that year.
- Compare the same test to last year. How has the athlete improved over the year?
- Compare test results to the projected goal. What actually happened on the testing day?

One rule to always remember is to decide what is important is each athlete's individual progress. Each athlete has to be able to progress at his or her own pace. Numbers are not important; it is how much improvement occurred that makes a difference.

Presenting Results to the Sport Coaches

If you are strength training athletes from several sports you need to keep the position or event coaches, head coaches, team trainers, or other interested individuals up-to-date with the test results. Inform each of them on their particular players, how they are progressing, and even how they compare with the rest of the team. Find out what each coach wants and how they want the results presented. Test results should be discussed with the coaches because they have ultimate responsibility for their athletes' success.

Posting Results for the Athletes

As soon as testing is completed, the results should be posted in the locker room or weight room where the athletes can see them.

Be concerned about peer pressure, which can have positive or negative effects. Some athletes react favorably to having their results posted. Others might react negatively and withdraw. Be positive in your approach; never humiliate the athletes.

The results can be posted alphabetically or best to worst; by sport, position, age, exercise, or season; you might post team averages, position averages, percent improvements for each athlete; you might post a list of the top 10 by exercise or total exercises, or a most improved list, to name a few. The way you post the results depends on your own preference.

Comparing Results to Goals

After you have tested the athletes you may want to compare the results to the goals that were set before the cycle started. You may be disappointed to find that some athletes did not improve or achieve their goals. Any of the following reasons could explain their failure to succeed.

- Goals were set too high. Many times it is quite difficult to predict how much an athlete will improve.
- The athletes did not work hard enough. Most of the time you can tell if this is the case by workout intensity, attendance, athlete motivation, and test results.
- The test may not have motivated the athlete. Some athletes love to train but do not get motivated by testing. You must make sure the athlete has incentives to test at his or her best. See chapter 5, "Motivation."
- The athlete may have trained improperly, and the tests show problems with the program.
- The test may have been given at the wrong time. If it is given the day before the first day of practice, the athlete may not want to excel in the weight room. Or, the test may have been done after a very hard workout, and the athlete was tired.
- The athlete may have had minor injuries and was not able to complete the training requirements.
- The athlete's strength level may be very high, which means significant continuous progress was hard to achieve. At this level some might not show any progress at the end of a cycle. This is normal.
- Some athletes, no matter how hard they work or how good the program, will not be as strong or make gains as big as others. They are not as genetically gifted. Always keep in mind this "genetic factor."

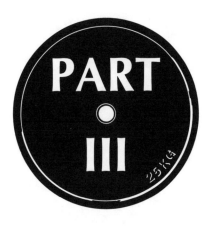

STRENGTH TRAINING
EXERCISES

CHAPTER
10

Core Exercises
for the Upper Body

Upper-body strength is important in all sports, especially contact sports. Many athletes and coaches incorrectly associate upper-body strength exclusively with bench-press strength. In reality the bench press is just one of many upper-body exercises. The bench press will develop chest strength, but there is more to upper-body strength than just strong pecs. Contrary to popular belief, the most important aspect of upper-body strength is shoulder strength. The upper back is also very important, and this area is sometimes neglected. Therefore, the athlete should be concerned with developing the whole upper body, not just a specific area. At times, emphasis can be placed on a certain area depending on the sport, but total upper-body strength is still desirable. To achieve this the athlete must perform a variety of upper-body exercises. In this chapter I will present a variety of exercises aimed at improving total upper-body strength.

The following safety considerations and training aid suggestions should be followed for each of the exercises in this chapter.

- Instruct your athletes always to follow proper breathing techniques. These are outlined in each exercise.
- See that your athletes use the recommended number of spotters and proper spotting techniques.
- Be sure your athletes are using a weight that can be handled without sacrificing technique.
- Tell your athletes that the use of belts is not necessary when performing upper-body exercises. For many athletes these merely serve as psychological support.
- Inform your athletes that the use of wrist wraps or tape is not recommended. They prevent the wrists from being strengthened to their fullest.
- Center the bar on the rack and balance the same amount of weight on each side.
- Place plates in the correct sequence and use collars.

BENCH PRESS

Ask athletes how strong they are and they will tell you how much they can bench press. This is because most athletes think the bench press is *the* measure of strength. The bench press is a simple exercise that produces a strong-looking chest and is often mistakenly thought of as the measure of a better athlete. In fact, the bench press is only a foundational exercise for developing and strengthening the upper-body muscles (i.e., chest [pecs], shoulders [deltoids], and back of the arms [triceps]). It should always be combined with other upper-body exercises, never used as the sole upper-body developer.

The bench press is not commonly thought of as a dangerous lift. It is, in fact, one of the most dangerous exercises performed because the weight is moved directly over the face and throat. The athlete must be alert and concentrate fully on the technique of the exercise.

It is important to control the weight on the down phase to protect the rib cage and the fragile muscles and ligaments in that area. The athlete should never bounce the bar off the chest or use a towel to bounce the bar on. The athlete should touch the bar lightly to the chest and immediately begin the upward drive.

Spotting Technique

A spotter should always be used. He or she should be standing behind the bar, close to the athlete's head, and preferably elevated. The elevation provides leverage. The spotter's hands should be spaced evenly, very close to the bar, and be able to grab the bar quickly to balance it and prevent serious injury. If the athlete cannot complete the lift on the upward movement, the spotter should quickly get his or her hands under the bar and pull the weight back up to the supports. The spotter can also provide a lift-off if it is needed (see chapter 4, ''Weight Room Safety''). Usually only one spotter is needed; if heavy weights are used, however, three are necessary, one behind the athlete and one on each side of the bar.

Exercise Technique

Breathing

The athlete unracks the bar, inhales, and holds his or her breath while lowering the bar. Then the athlete exhales *slowly* all the way to the top of the upward push. Or, alternatively, the bar is unracked and positioned first. The athlete inhales while lowering the bar and exhales *slowly* while pushing the bar up.

Positioning the Body

The athlete lies on his or her back with head, back, and buttocks firmly on the bench. The lower back should have no more than a natural arch (Figure 10.1).

The legs are placed on each side of the bench with knees bent and feet planted firmly and flat on the floor, pointing forward or turned slightly outward. This aids in stability and keeps the body tight during the exercise.

In this position the bar in the rack should be directly above the lifter's eyes.

Grip and Hand Placement

Using the knurlings on the bar as a guide, the athlete's hands should be placed slightly wider than shoulder width apart. Athletes with longer arms might use a wider grip; those with shorter arms will use a closer grip. Usually the athlete will use a grip slightly wider than shoulder width, which will cause the bar to move in a more linear path, while a closer grip will give the bar an arced path. The movement of the bar, however,

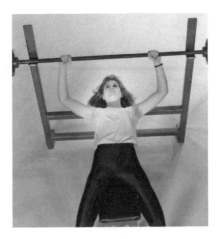

Figure 10.1   Correct positioning for the bench press.

is not critical in the exercise performance. The grip is a matter of individual preference and should be comfortable (Figure 10.1).

The grip also determines the amount of emphasis placed on certain muscles. To develop the total chest area the grip should be just slightly wider than the shoulders. This will work the chest muscles more. However, if the grip is extremely wide the range of motion decreases, which places less initial stress on the muscles and is an inefficient way of getting stronger. A closer grip puts more emphasis on the shoulders and triceps. Often the sport and position an athlete plays determines the width of the bench press grip. For example, a discus thrower might use a wider grip than an offensive or defensive lineman.

The athlete should use a firm grip with thumbs wrapped around the bar (Figure 10.2). The wrists should not be hyperextended. This places too much stress on the forearm and wrists.

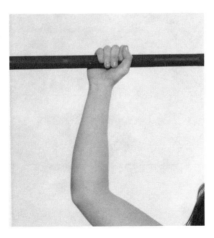

Figure 10.2   Grip for the bench press.

Unracking the Bar

The athlete should push the bar off the supports in a strong, controlled manner. The arms extend and elbows partially lock (Figure 10.3). Most of the pressure should be on the shoulders when the arms are straight.

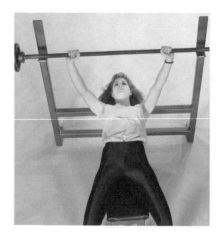

Figure 10.3   Unracking the bar.

The bar should move forward, slightly away from the supports, and should rest somewhere over the top of the sternum.

Down Phase

The athlete slowly lowers the bar down to the chest (Figures 10.4a and b). The bar should be straight over the wrists, forearms, and elbows. Moving the bar slowly works the negative part of the lift, the eccentric contraction. The bar does not necessarily move in a straight line. Because of the way muscle joints work (in a rotation) it will move in a slight curve.

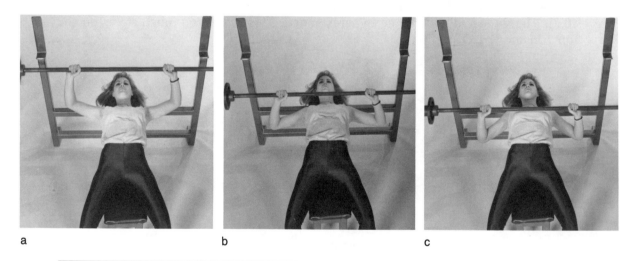

a   b   c

Figure 10.4   The down phase.

At the bottom the bar should lightly touch the chest near the nipples (Figure 10.4c). Also, at this point, the elbows should be out and under the bar (Figure 10.5). If lowered below the nipple line it can cause injury to the xiphoid process, which is a cartilage-type bone of the lower part of the sternum. Never let the athlete bounce the bar. Touch lightly, stop momentarily, and push off.

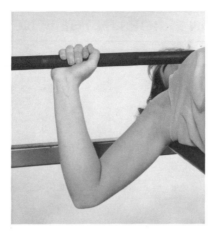

Figure 10.5   The elbows should be out and under the bar during the down phase.

Upward Phase

In this phase all the muscles involved with the bench press contract to push the bar upward (Figure 10.6a). The push should be forceful but under control and not jerky. The athlete should push the bar back to the starting position above the sternum, making sure to extend the arms fully. The athlete should feel "tight-strong" throughout the movement (Figure 10.6b).

When your athletes rack the bar do not let them slam the bar backward against the bench supports.

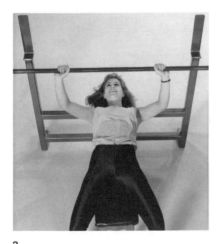

a

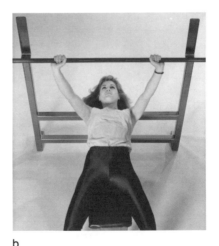

b

Figure 10.6   The upward phase.

COMMON ERRORS IN THE BENCH PRESS

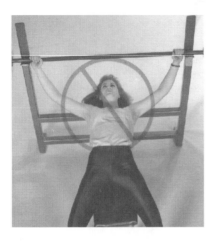

Figure 10.7 The athlete should not use a grip much wider than shoulder width.

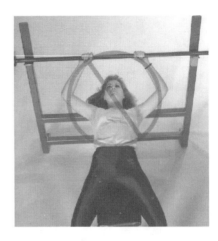

Figure 10.8 The grip should not be too close.

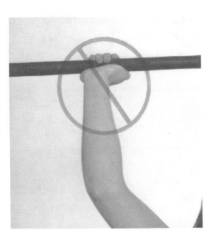

Figure 10.9 The thumbs should not be under the bar but around the bar to prevent it from slipping out of the hands.

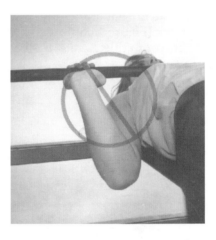

Figure 10.10 The elbows should not be close to the body and away from the bar.

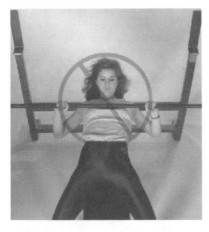

Figure 10.11 Athletes should not bounce the bar or raise their heads off the bench.

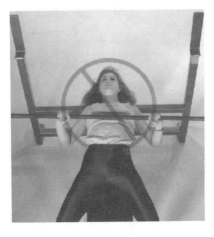

Figure 10.12 The bar should not be lowered near the abdominal area.

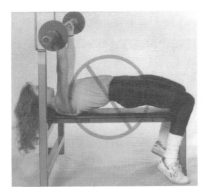

Figure 10.13   When the athlete pushes the weight up, the hips should not be lifted off the bench.

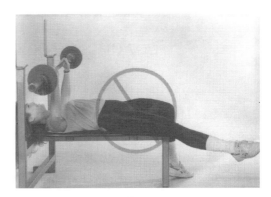

Figure 10.14   During the entire exercise the body stays stationary and the legs should not move or extend.

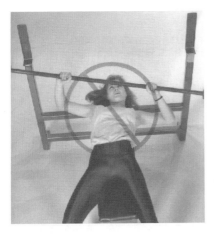

Figure 10.15   The bar should not be pushed up unevenly. This can be an indication of muscle imbalance.

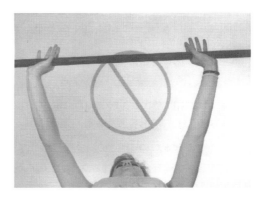

Figure 10.16   The firm grip on the bar should not be released until the bar is securely racked.

COACH'S CHECKLIST: BENCH PRESS

☐ Bar loaded evenly, collars in place

☐ Athlete lies on bench, eyes under bar

☐ Hands placed evenly on bar

☐ Grip slightly wider than shoulder width

☐ Thumbs around bar, wrists locked

☐ Body and head rest on bench throughout exercise

☐ Legs placed on each side of bench

☐ Feet flat on floor

☐ Bar lifted off rack in controlled manner

☐ Bar stabilized over upper chest, arms straight, elbows locked, and grip tight

☐ Momentary stop

☐ Bar lowered slowly to chest in controlled manner, close to nipples

☐ Momentary stop

☐ Bar driven up to starting position

☐ Head and hips kept on bench

☐ Athlete should not arch, twist body, or move feet

☐ Bar returned to rack in controlled manner

INCLINE PRESS

The incline press is a great exercise for strengthening the upper body, especially the shoulder area. It is similar to the military press in the angles used and the muscles worked (i.e., shoulder [deltoids], chest [pecs], back of arm [triceps], upper back [traps]). I prefer the incline over the military press because the hips and back are supported, which eliminates unnecessary stress on the lower back, and enables the athlete to lift more weight.

This exercise can be performed with various equipment, most commonly an Olympic bar with an incline bench. A preferred angle for the back rest of the incline bench is 40 to 45 degrees. Many inclines are built at 35 degrees or less. But at less than 35 degrees the exercise is too similar to the bench press. By using a greater incline, more shoulder work is done.

Spotting Technique

Spotters should always be used in this exercise. For leverage, the spotter stands on a platform behind the lifter. Most modern equipment has built-in spotter platforms. If no platform exists the spotter should stand on a utility bench, close to the athlete, with hands near the bar. If the athlete cannot complete the upward movement the spotter should quickly get his or her hands under the bar and pull the weight back up to the supports. The spotter can also provide a lift-off as in the bench press if needed (see chapter 4, "Weight Room Safety"). Usually only one spotter is needed; if near-maximum weights are used, however, three are necessary, one behind the athlete and one on each side.

Exercise Technique

Breathing

The athlete unracks the bar, inhales, and holds the breath while lowering the bar. He or she exhales *slowly* all the way to the top of the upward push. Or, alternatively, the athlete unracks the bar and positions it first. Then the athlete inhales while lowering the bar and exhales *slowly* while pushing the bar up.

Positioning the Body

The athlete sits with hips, back, shoulders, and head resting against the bench. Legs are to the side with knees bent and feet flat on the floor. Keeping the legs to the side maintains a stable position (Figure 10.17).

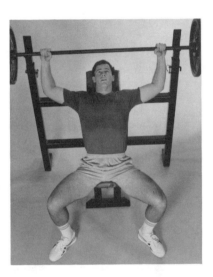

Figure 10.17   Correct positioning for the incline press.

Grip and Hand Placement

Using the knurlings as a guide, the athlete places the hands a comfortable distance apart with thumbs around the bar (Figure 10.17). The normal placement is slightly wider than shoulder width apart. Taller athletes will have a wider grip; shorter athletes will have a narrower grip. Usually the grip distance is similar to the one used in the bench press.

Down Phase

The athlete pushes the bar off the support and keeps it at arm's length with the elbows locked. The weight is kept directly over the wrists and elbows without hyperextending the wrists. The bar rests high over the eyes (Figure 10.18a).

As the athlete slowly lowers the bar, the elbows are kept out, creating a 90 degree angle with the torso (Figure 10.18b). The athlete lowers the bar to the top of the sternum, very close to the face (Figure 10.18c).

Do not allow athletes to bounce the bar off the chest. There is little muscle in this area of the chest, and it would be very uncomfortable and dangerous to bounce the

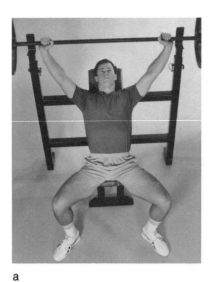
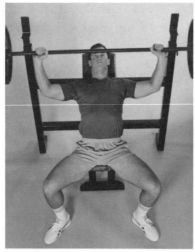
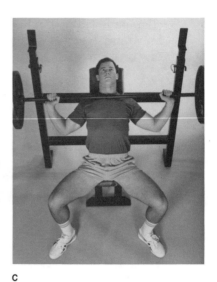

a   b   c

Figure 10.18 The down phase.

bar at that position. The bar should touch the chest lightly, and the athlete should immediately begin the upward movement.

Upward Phase

Keeping head down on the bench, body tight, and elbows out to the side, the athlete should push the bar smoothly (with no jerky movements) straight up over the face until the arms are fully extended. It should feel almost as if the bar is being pushed backward (Figures 10.19a, b).

During the entire movement the athlete should focus on the ceiling, not the bar. The athlete should track the bar with peripheral vision.

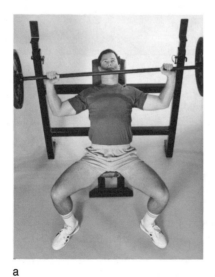
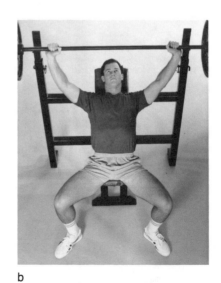

a   b

Figure 10.19 The upward phase.

COMMON ERRORS IN THE INCLINE PRESS

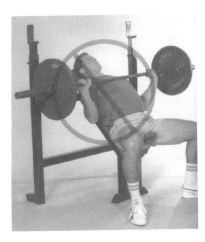

Figure 10.20   The bar should not be lowered too low onto the chest or push the elbows close to the body.

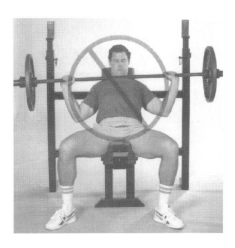

Figure 10.21   The head should not be raised off the bench.

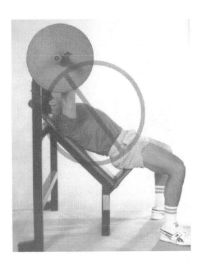

Figure 10.22   The hips should not be raised off the bench.

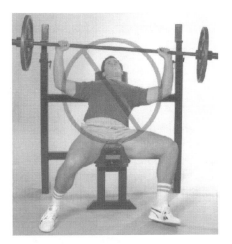

Figure 10.23   When pushing the weight upward, the athlete should not twist, pushing the bar unevenly.

COACH'S CHECKLIST: INCLINE PRESS

☐ Bar loaded evenly, collars in place
☐ Grip slightly wider than shoulder width
☐ Thumbs around bar
☐ Athlete seated comfortably, hips and back secure on bench
☐ Legs placed on each side of bench, feet flat on floor
☐ Head on bench
☐ Bar lifted off rack in controlled manner
☐ Momentary stop
☐ Bar lowered to top of chest, close to chin
☐ Elbows out, forming 90-degree angle
☐ Bar lowered almost in straight line
☐ Bar stopped momentarily and moved up in straight line
☐ Body tight, hips down, feet flat on floor throughout exercise
☐ Arms locked but without jamming the bar
☐ Bar returned to rack in controlled manner

BEHIND-THE-NECK PRESS

The behind-the-neck press is the only major press that requires the athlete to push weight behind the head. The exercise helps strengthen the upper-back muscles and provides a balance to the bench press. This exercise also avoids rounded shoulders caused by excessive bench-press work. Specifically, it trains the shoulders (deltoids), arms (triceps), and upper back (trapezius). This exercise also provides necessary shoulder flexibility.

The behind-the-neck press can be done from a standing or seated position. The technique is the same regardless of the apparatus used. In the seated position the upper-back muscles are isolated. In the standing position, the athlete might have a tendency to use his or her legs to lift the weight. Because the weight is pushed over the head, the athlete should wear a belt for lower-back and abdominal stability.

Spotting Technique

A spotter should always be used. For leverage, the spotter should stand in an elevated position behind the bar and close to the athlete's head. Usually only one spotter is needed; if heavy weights are used, however, three are necessary, one behind the athlete and one on each side.

Exercise Technique

Breathing

The athlete unracks the bar, inhales, and holds the breath while lowering the bar. He or she exhales *slowly* all the way to the top of the upward push. Or, alternatively, the athlete unracks the bar and positions it first. The athlete inhales while lowering the bar and exhales *slowly* while pushing the bar up.

Grip and Hand Placement

The grip is slightly wider than shoulder width, thumbs around the bar, elbows straight under the bar, and wrists locked. Do not allow athletes to hyperextend their wrists or move their elbows forward.

The athlete sits with back straight, preferably supported, thighs parallel to the floor, and feet flat on the floor. The head should be facing straight ahead. The exercise begins with the weight on the athlete's upper back and shoulders (Figure 10.24).

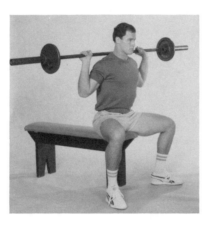

Figure 10.24 Correct positioning for the behind-the-neck press.

Upward Phase

During the upward drive the athlete's back should not arch or twist. The back should remain straight and the head forward (Figure 10.25a). The athlete must push the bar straight up, feeling almost as if pushing the bar backward, not over the head. The elbows are kept out and the bar is pushed until the arms are fully extended (Figure 10.25b, c). It is a little easier to do the exercise by leaning the head forward a little,

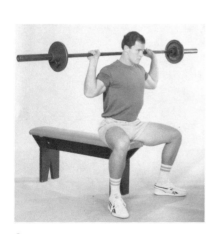
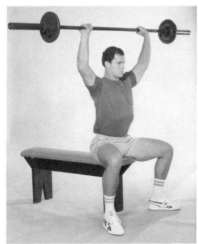
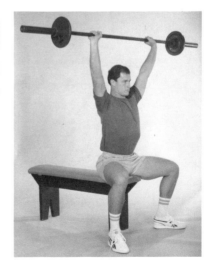

a   b   c

Figure 10.25 The upward phase.

leaving room for the bar to go up and down in a straight line. The bar should not move in a curved path. The athlete should not jam the bar but should stop momentarily at the top.

Down Phase

From the top position the athlete lowers the bar very gradually as in any other press. This part is the eccentric contraction, an important part of strength training. The elbows stay all the way out so the upper arm is on the same plane as the torso. The bar lowers straight down to the neck area close to the ears, but not all the way to the traps (Figure 10.26a). At this point the athlete stops momentarily, then pushes the bar back up in a straight line (Figure 10.26b). At the top the torso and arms should be straight and the bar held high overhead.

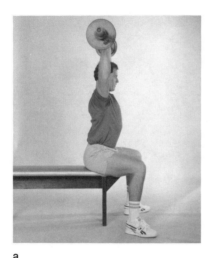
a

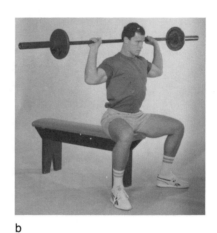
b

Figure 10.26   The down phase.

COMMON ERRORS IN THE BEHIND-THE-NECK PRESS

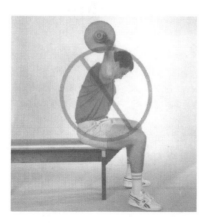

Figure 10.27   During the upward drive the back must not be rounded.

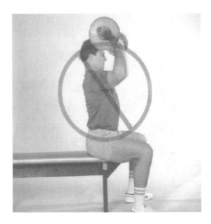

Figure 10.28   Because of poor shoulder flexibility the athlete might have a tendency to drive the bar and elbows forward.

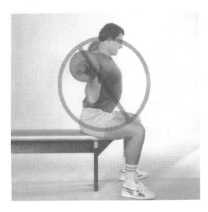

Figure 10.29 In the down phase, do not lower the bar too low and put excessive pressure on the shoulders.

COACH'S CHECKLIST: BEHIND-THE-NECK PRESS

- ☐ Bar loaded evenly, collars in place
- ☐ Bar placed high on upper back
- ☐ Hands placed shoulder width apart
- ☐ Thumbs around bar
- ☐ Wrists straight, locked tight
- ☐ Elbows under bar
- ☐ Athlete seated with back straight, head up
- ☐ Feet to sides, flat on floor
- ☐ Bar pushed straight overhead
- ☐ Arms extended to full length
- ☐ Momentary stop
- ☐ Bar lowered slowly to ears
- ☐ Momentary stop
- ☐ Bar pushed upward again
- ☐ Bar always moved in straight line

CHAPTER

11

Core Exercises for the Lower Body

The importance of upper-body strength can vary from one sport to another, but lower-body strength is critical to all sports. Lower-body strength lies mainly in the hips, because this is the center of gravity, where all movements start. It is also the most powerful part of the body and contains the largest muscles. Power in this area helps the athlete run faster, jump higher, and hit harder. Improvement in lower-body strength can be directly related to improved athletic performance.

Lower-body injuries can usually be attributed to muscular imbalance and poor flexibility. The most common injury in the lower body is a pulled hamstring. Every coach is concerned with this particular injury. The next most common injury occurs in the knee joint, which is very unstable because it consists of two bones, sitting one atop the other, with only ligaments and tendons holding them together. This vulnerability is especially noticeable in contact sports such as football. Strengthening the muscles, tendons, and ligaments that surround the knee joint will reduce the occurrence of these injuries. Exercises such as the squat, walking lunges, and leg press not only strengthen the knee and hip-joint area but also increase flexibility.

The following safety precautions and lifting aid suggestions should be used any time lower-body exercises are done.

- Remind athletes to use proper breathing at all times. Athletes should never hold their breath through the entire movement because this could cause dizziness. In each exercise I explain proper breathing techniques.
- Use the recommended number of spotters and the proper spotting techniques, also explained in the exercise technique sections.
- Do not allow athletes to use knee wraps or lifting suits. These may permit the use of heavier weight, but they inhibit strength development at the knee and hip joints.
- Allow athletes to use a lifting belt if desired.
- Do not place a pad or towel around the bar. This can cause the bar to roll off the shoulders.

- Instruct athletes always to wear shoes that lend firm ankle support and have hard soles—tennis shoes, for example. Because they lack lateral support, running shoes are not recommended.
- Center the bar on the rack and balance the same amount of weight on each side.
- Place plates in the correct sequence (heavier plates first followed by lighter ones).

BACK SQUAT

The back or barbell squat is often referred to as the "king of exercises" for valid reasons. I believe no other exercise trains the legs and hips as well as this squat does. Proper technique and intensity are necessary for the exercise to be beneficial. It should be performed with a full range of motion (down, parallel to the floor, and up to a vertical position) for optimum strength gains and to maintain or gain hip flexibility. Intensity will vary with the athlete's sport and maturity.

Because of the high chance of injury, especially at the knee joint, some coaches think squatting is not worth the risk. Sufficient evidence exists indicating that the knee joint is actually strengthened through squatting. The exercise makes the muscles around the knee joint stronger. In my opinion, the squat is the most important lower-body strength exercise for athletes.

The exercise trains the powerful explosive muscles of the lower body (quadriceps, hamstrings, groin, hips, and lower back) used in running, jumping, and throwing. It is also a great time saver because with this single exercise the athlete can strengthen the entire lower body.

All athletes should squat using a safe apparatus like a wide power rack with safety catch (squat inside rack) or a regular step rack with a safety bar at the bottom.

Some athletes cannot squat to parallel position and keep their heels flat on the floor. This is usually the result of poor hip and ankle flexibility. Do not try to remedy the problem by putting a board or plates under an athlete's heels. This will do nothing to improve flexibility and will teach athletes to squat incorrectly. This "remedy" causes the body to shift forward and put too much pressure on the knees. Be patient; work on proper stance and flexibility by using light loads.

The use of chairs or boxes to squat on can also be very dangerous. These kinds of apparatus are usually used to teach sitting back and reaching proper depth. The athlete should never sit on a box or chair and relax with weight on the shoulders. This puts a lot of pressure on the lower back. If the athlete uses these apparatus, he or she should touch them lightly and drive up. I believe the athlete should "feel" the movement and take the time to do it correctly without the use of such apparatus.

Spotting Technique

All squat workouts should be supervised by at least two spotters (one on each side of the bar). If the load is heavy, a third spotter should stand behind the squatter. Spotters should never touch the bar unless the athlete needs assistance. Most of the assistance will be needed at the bottom position on the way up. If the spotters notice the athlete is losing control or technique and cannot drive the bar up alone, they should automatically intervene by grabbing the bar and assisting the lifter in racking the bar. Do not let the athlete's ego cause him or her to do the exercise incorrectly and take the chance of getting hurt.

Exercise Technique

Breathing

The athlete should inhale at the top of the squat, go down holding the breath, and exhale on the way up. Athletes may find it easier to do most of the exhaling after passing the sticking point (half way in upward drive).

The Start

The athlete's hands should be spaced evenly on the bar so that when the bar is racked on the shoulders the weight will be evenly distributed. A wide grip with the thumbs wrapped around the bar is preferred.

Under the bar, the athlete's knees are bent, chest out, back straight with a slight arch at the waist, and hips directly under the bar.

The bar should be racked comfortably on the upper back and shoulders (Figure 11.1a). Many athletes make the mistake of placing the bar too high near the neck, which results in discomfort or even pain. Others may rack the bar too low, making it easy for the bar to slip off.

While keeping firm pressure against the bar the athlete lifts the bar off the rack. At this time, all the muscles of the torso and hips should be contracted. The bar should be lifted in a controlled movement by extending at the knees. Do not let the athlete jam his or her shoulders upward against the bar from a relaxed position.

The athlete takes only one step back, bringing both legs together. The athlete should not take more than one step back.

The body should be straight, with head up and arms under the bar to help with stability (Figure 11.1b).

Feet should be slightly wider than shoulder width apart, toes pointing slightly out to the side (Figure 11.1c). This stance is ideal for athletes who want good overall lower-body strength. The athlete should not use a "bodybuilder" stance where the legs are too close together and the toes are pointing straight ahead. This stance could lead to knee problems. The athlete should also not use a "power lifter" stance where the legs are too far apart and the feet are pointing too far to the side.

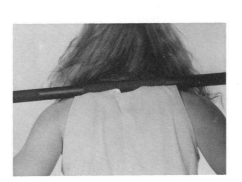
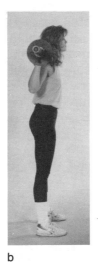
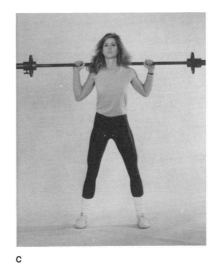

a   b   c

Figure 11.1   The start.

Downward Movement

The athlete should begin the descent by bending at the hips first, *not* at the knees (Figure 11.2a). This is where most knee problems occur. The athlete should not lower his or her hips straight down, pushing the knees forward past the toes. The knees should not go past the toes very much in this exercise. There should be very little pressure placed on the knees (Figure 11.2b). I think you can see clearly how the squat has had a bad reputation as an exercise that causes knee injuries. It is improper squatting, however, *not* the exercise itself, that causes knee problems.

The athlete should bend at the hips and sit back slowly, under control, to a parallel position. Never let the athlete "free-fall" to the bottom position. Avoid excessive

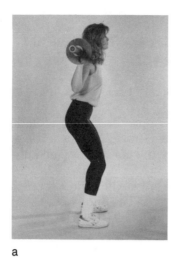
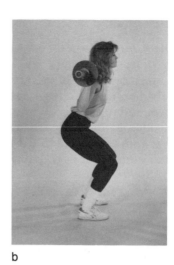

a   b

Figure 11.2   The downward movement is started by bending at the hips first.

forward lean of the torso by telling the athlete to keep the bar over the hips as much as possible. The more the athlete leans forward, the less the hips and legs get strengthened. The lower back is kept locked and tight.

The Bottom Position

The athlete should descend until the thighs are parallel to the floor (Figure 11.3). Remember, all exercises should be performed with a full range of motion, so it is very important that the athlete go to a full parallel position in this exercise. Partial squats lead to overdevelopment of the quadriceps at the expense of the hamstring. This imbalance can contribute to knee and hamstring injuries. When the athlete goes to parallel position, all the muscles of the legs and hips get strengthened. It is better for the athlete to use less weight and do the exercise fully than to use more weight and do only partial squats. The athlete will also gain hip flexibility by doing the exercise with a full range of motion. Going beyond parallel is not necessary.

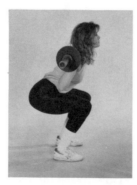

Figure 11.3   The bottom position.

Do not allow your athlete to bounce at the bottom of the squat. Bouncing at the bottom can injure the connective tissue of the knee. It may allow the athlete to use more weight but does little for building real strength. When the athlete bounces, the weight is lifted by momentum, not strength.

The athlete should not lean forward at the bottom of this exercise. The back should be straight, with knees over the toes, elbows under the bar, head up, chest out, and feet flat on the floor. Lack of hip and ankle flexibility can cause the athlete to squat up on the toes. Weight should be evenly distributed on the balls and heels of the feet during the entire movement.

The Upward Movement

After reaching the parallel position and stopping momentarily, the athlete begins the ascent by pushing with the legs and driving the hips up under the bar (Figure 11.4a). The athlete might think of pushing the feet through the floor. The push should be forceful but always under control. Once past the sticking point, the athlete should slow down so as not to bounce the bar off the shoulders at the top. Through the ascent, the athlete must maintain a tight torso and a straight, upright back and keep the shoulders higher than the hips (Figure 11.4b). If these points are not observed, unnecessary pressure is placed on the lower back, which could result in injury.

Some athletes have a bad habit of pushing the knees in while pushing up. Leg power is lost when the knees come together, and too much pressure is placed on the inside ligaments of the knee. It is important to keep the knees out over the feet when pushing the bar up.

At the top, the bar should not be jammed so that the weights rattle. After passing the sticking point, the athlete should not put as much pressure on the bar and should come to a slow stop. When the lift is completed the torso and hips should not relax but keep a strong, tight feeling until the bar is racked (Figure 11.4c).

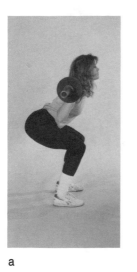 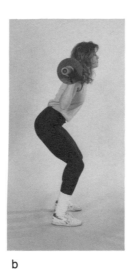 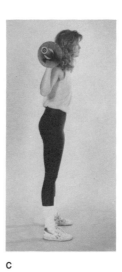

a   b   c

Figure 11.4   The upward movement.

Racking the Bar

When the lift is completed, make sure your athlete racks the bar correctly. Athletes should never move toward the rack until the lift is completed. From the standing position the athlete should step forward in a controlled manner, first one foot, then the other. Now the athlete should be standing very close to the rack with the bar over the safety pins. By bending at the hips and keeping the head up and body straight the athlete slowly lowers the bar onto the rack. When the bar rests on the pins the athlete can move out from under the bar.

COMMON ERRORS IN THE BACK SQUAT

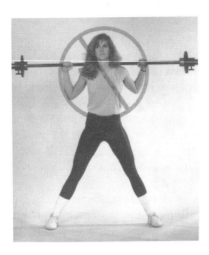

Figure 11.5 The athlete should not use a very wide stance when squatting.

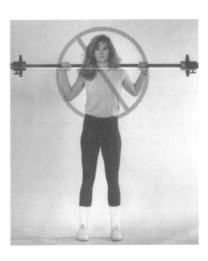

Figure 11.6 A very narrow stance will put excessive pressure on the knees.

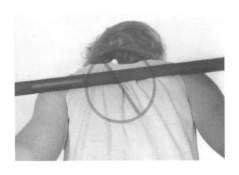

Figure 11.7 The bar should not be placed too low on the back.

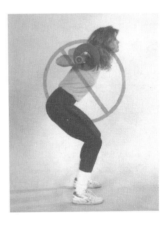

Figure 11.8 The elbows should not be out and back.

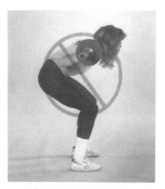

Figure 11.9 The athlete should never squat with a rounded back.

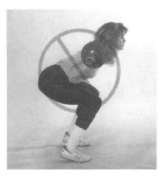

Figure 11.10 Some athletes have a tendency to go up on their toes while squatting.

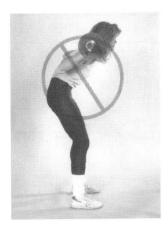

Figure 11.11   In the upward drive, the upper back does not relax.

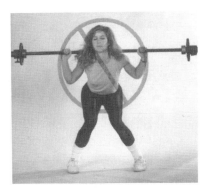

Figure 11.12   Knees should not be pushed inward on the drive up.

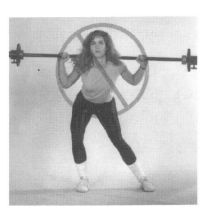

Figure 11.13   Because of muscle imbalance, some athletes have a tendency to shift body weight in the upward drive.

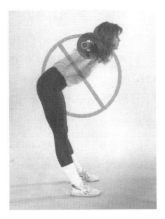

Figure 11.14   The athlete should not extend the legs before the upper back.

COACH'S CHECKLIST: BACK SQUAT

☐ Bar on rack is approximately chest height
☐ Hands spaced evenly and slightly wider than shoulder width apart
☐ Bar rests across traps and back of shoulders
☐ Chest up and out
☐ Head up
☐ Shoulder blades pushed together
☐ Torso straight and tight
☐ Athlete takes one step back
☐ Feet shoulder width apart
☐ Toes slightly out, feet flat on floor
☐ Hips bend first
☐ Knees bend and stay over toes
☐ Athlete sits back over heels
☐ Athlete squats to parallel position with tops of thighs parallel to floor
☐ Momentary stop
☐ Bar driven up to starting position
☐ Hips kept under bar
☐ Knees kept out
☐ Weight kept centered
☐ Bar comes to slow stop at top

LEG PRESS

The leg press is an excellent exercise for strengthening the lower body. The simplicity of the exercise also allows the athlete to use relatively heavy weights. It is one of the safer exercises because weight is supported by the machine. Since it does not require a great deal of teaching and supervision it is especially good for younger athletes. For more advanced athletes the leg press is used for auxiliary work. Better lower-body strength is gained by doing squats along with the leg press.

The purpose of the leg press is to develop the lower body by extending the knees and hips. The quads, the hams, and the glutes are being worked. The hip angle used in the leg press will dictate how much work the hips and upper part of the hamstrings get. If the angle is tighter (knees close to the chest) the athlete has to give a longer push; therefore, groin muscles and the upper hamstrings work harder.

One drawback is that because the hips are not fully extended, the exercise limits the development of the big muscles in the hips and the lower back. The lower back is completely rested, so very little back work is done.

The leg press is a very popular exercise because of the versatility of the equipment used. Many different types of leg press machines are made, allowing athletes to be seated or to lie back on the floor or pronated at a variety of angles. The angles of the different leg presses will vary the results somewhat, but the general work concept remains the same. Whatever the style of the equipment, the technique is similar.

Spotting Technique

Spotters are not generally used in this exercise.

Exercise Technique

Breathing

The athlete inhales at the bottom or while the weight is lowered and exhales while driving the weight upward. Athletes should not hold their breath while performing several repetitions but should inhale and exhale for each repetition.

Some athletes have been known to get headaches or black out while doing this exercise. This is due to improper breathing technique: Athletes are holding their breath for too long. Proper breathing technique should be used in each repetition.

Positioning

In the two most common types of leg press the athlete either sits with back supported and presses forward at an angle or takes a supine (lying down) position and presses straight up. In either position the feet are placed approximately shoulder width apart and the athlete presses with the balls and heels of the feet, toes pointed slightly out. The athlete should never press with the toes: Excessive pressure is placed on the knees and feet, which can result in knee irritation or injury. By pressing with the balls and heels of the feet the stress is channeled into the hip area, which can sustain more stress. Some machines have pedals that do not allow variation in the width at which athletes can place their feet. The machine should allow athletes to vary the width. A taller athlete will need wider foot placement than a shorter athlete.

Pressing Angle

For a good pressing angle, the knees should be flexed at about 90 degrees (Figure 11.15). The athlete may reduce the angle to 60 degrees. This will provide more of a stretch, and more of the lower-body muscles will be involved. This will put the hamstrings and quads into a pre-stretch. The hips are also put into a pre-stretch, and therefore the athlete will create more power.

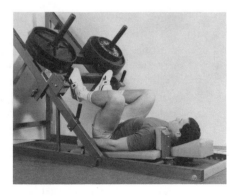

Figure 11.15   Correct pressing angle.

Raising the Weight

The back should stay firmly on the back support, with the hands grasping the handles for stability. The head should be kept down. The whole body is tight. The athlete pushes forward forcefully, in a controlled manner (Figure 11.16a), and exerts pressure all the way forward until the legs are fully extended (Figure 11.16b). Make sure the athlete gives a strong, forward push and does not lose control, causing the feet to slip off the apparatus. Up top, the legs are extended but not fully locked.

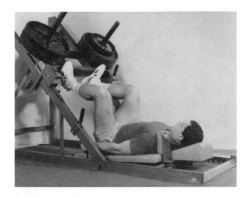 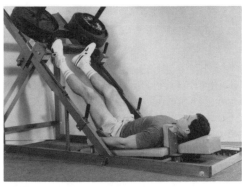

a   b

Figure 11.16   Correct technique for raising the weight.

Lowering the Weight

At the top the athlete pauses momentarily and slowly lowers the weight to the starting position. The weight platform should barely touch the support before the next press is begun. The weight platform should not come all the way down and stop. The athlete must maintain tension to start the next rep and should not bounce the weight platform at the bottom to gain momentum.

COMMON ERRORS IN THE LEG PRESS

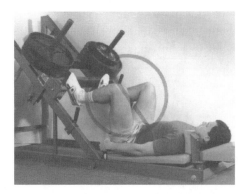 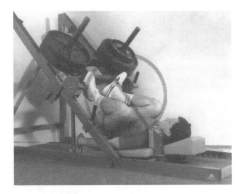

Figure 11.17   The body should not be too far away from the moving carriage.

Figure 11.18   The body should not be too close to the moving carriage, making the hips come off the back support.

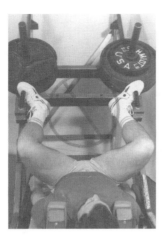

Figure 11.19   The feet and knees should not point out too far.

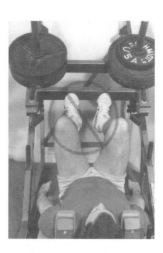

Figure 11.20   The athlete should not put all the weight on the toes but on the balls of the feet.

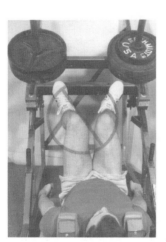

Figure 11.21   The knees should not be pushed inward when pressing the weight.

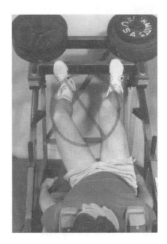

Figure 11.22   The body should not twist in the pressing movement.

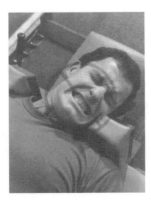

Figure 11.23   The athlete should not tighten up the head and neck when performing the exercise.

COACH'S CHECKLIST: LEG PRESS

☐ Back and head supported
☐ Feet placed on leg press, approximately shoulder width apart
☐ Toes pointed slightly outward
☐ Pressure on balls and heels of feet
☐ Knee angle reaches 90 to 60 degrees
☐ Hips flat against bench
☐ Hands to side for stability
☐ Athlete presses forcefully to top position
☐ Knees kept pointing out
☐ Head stays down
☐ Legs extend fully
☐ Knees partially locked
☐ Athlete stops momentarily
☐ Weight lowered slowly back to starting position
☐ Weight not bounced at bottom

DEAD LIFT

The dead lift is one of the best tests of overall body strength. The dead lift is often associated with power lifting: The competitive power lifter tries to lift as much weight as possible. This can give the wrong impression to athletes and coaches. The dead lift should be used as a training exercise, not as a competition. Like any other exercise, proper technique and intensity must be used.

Because young athletes, especially at the high school level, need raw total-body strength and muscle mass, this exercise is good for them. The dead lift provides a good base for the more advanced, more explosive pulling exercises they will be doing as they mature. As athletes progress in strength and maturity they can eliminate the dead lift from their workouts and do more explosive exercises such as the power clean and high pulls.

The dead lift is a multijoint exercise involving the knees, hips, and to some degree the shoulders. This exercise trains all the muscles of the lower body: the quads, hamstrings, groin, hip flexors, gluteus maximus, lower-back erectors, and to a degree the trapezius and lats in the upper back. These are the same muscles used in sports that require thrusting of the hips and movements such as blocking, tackling, jumping, running, and throwing.

Spotting Technique

Spotters are not generally used in this exercise.

Exercise Technique

On first observation the lift technique appears simple. The athlete may think the only thing to do is to pick the weight up off the floor and stand up straight. Unfortunately, this kind of thinking can lead to injuries. Proper technique is of major importance to gaining maximum benefits and avoiding injury. The dead lift has several important stages that must be learned correctly.

There are two styles of dead lift, the conventional and the sumo style. For athletic training, the conventional style is best because it puts the legs, hips, and arms in an angle that is biomechanically similar to athletic movements. In the sumo style the legs are spread wide and the bar is grabbed in between the legs, not similar to athletic movements.

Breathing

The athlete inhales at the bottom when in the pulling stance. The breath is held during the entire pull to the top. At that time the athlete slowly exhales while lowering the bar to the starting position.

The Start

The athlete approaches the bar, placing his or her legs slightly less than shoulder width apart and toes pointing outward slightly. The athlete's feet are under the bar and the shins about two inches from the bar.

The athlete bends down and grabs the bar with both hands, one palm in and one palm out and thumbs around the bar (Figure 11.24a). This reverse grip allows the athlete to pull more weight. The thumb can be wrapped under the other fingers for a stronger grip, but this can be uncomfortable. The arms should be outside the legs and the grip shoulder width apart.

The back should be straight and parallel to the lower legs, and the thighs should be generally parallel to the floor. The back is kept straight throughout the movement and acts as a single lever with the fulcrum at the hips.

The athlete should be looking forward, head and shoulders squared over the bar. It helps to be focusing on an imaginary spot straight ahead throughout the movement. The arms should be kept straight (Figure 11.24b). The pulling is done with the legs, hips, and back, not the arms. Feet should be kept flat on the floor. As they are pulling the weight, athletes will feel as though they are trying to push their feet through the floor.

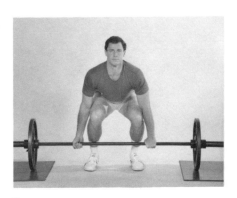
a

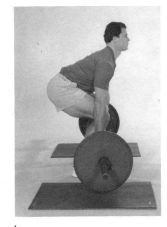
b

Figure 11.24   The start.

The Pull

The athlete must pull the bar slowly with no jerking movement, extending with the legs and keeping the back straight. The bar should be pulled very close to the body (right by the shins), and the athlete should move the knees back slightly so the bar can come up in a straight line. The sticking point is just under the knees (Figure 11.25a); this is the most strenuous part of the exercise. Past the knees the bar remains very close to the body (Figure 11.25b). The athlete pulls the bar straight up to a standing position and locks the knees (Figure 11.25c). The movement should not go any farther, stopping at the straight position (Figure 11.25d).

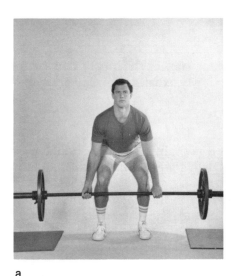

a

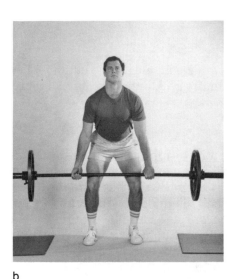

b

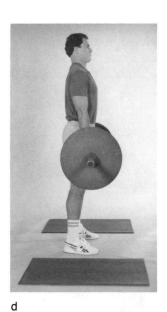

c   d

Figure 11.25 The pull.

Lowering the Bar

After the athlete stops momentarily at the top, he or she reverses the movement, slowly lowering the bar, bending at the hips and knees, and keeping the bar close to the body all the way to the floor. The bar should never be dropped to the floor but should be lowered under control

COMMON ERRORS IN THE DEAD LIFT

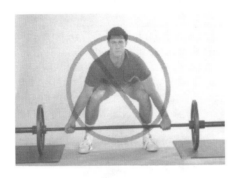

Figure 11.26 The stance and grip should not be excessively wide.

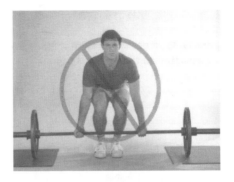

Figure 11.27 The feet should not be too close together.

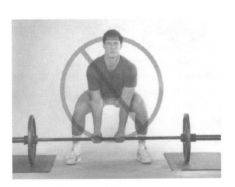

Figure 11.28 A "sumo" style grip is not recommended for athletes.

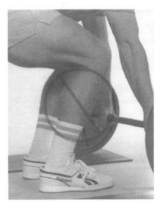

Figure 11.29 The bar should not be away from the body at the start of the exercise.

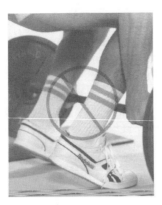

Figure 11.30   The athlete should not be up on the toes at the start of the exercise.

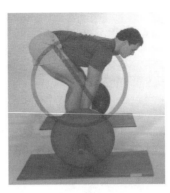

Figure 11.31   The hips should not be higher than the shoulders at the start.

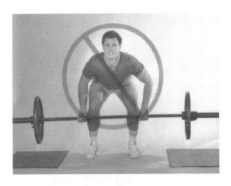

Figure 11.32   The bar should not be jammed off the ground at the start.

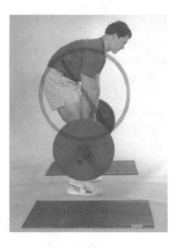

Figure 11.33   The exercise should not be executed with a round back.

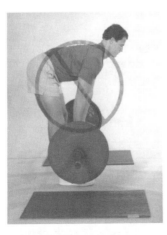

Figure 11.34   In the upward drive the legs should not be extended while the back is still bent forward.

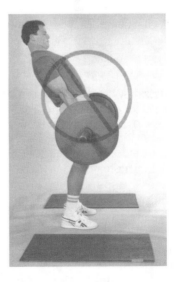

Figure 11.35   Up top, the athlete should not lean back excessively.

COACH'S CHECKLIST: DEAD LIFT

☐ Feet flat on floor
☐ Bar touching shins
☐ Hands placed outside legs
☐ Reverse grip, thumbs around bar
☐ Arms straight, elbows slightly touching legs
☐ Head up, chest up and out
☐ Back straight, shoulders back
☐ Hips low, below shoulders
☐ Thighs parallel to floor
☐ Bar lifted slowly
☐ Pulling done by extending legs and hips
☐ Arms remain straight
☐ Back remains straight
☐ Bar kept close to body
☐ Even pull to top
☐ Momentary stop at top
☐ Lower weight slowly
☐ Bar placed on floor

WALKING LUNGE

Most lower-body exercises work both legs simultaneously, but lunges require the athlete to work one leg at a time. Because of this, lunges stretch and strengthen certain hip and groin muscles like no other exercise can. Lunges work the same muscles as the squat and leg press but place more emphasis in the groin and at the top of the hamstring.

It is a great advantage to strength train one leg at a time because so many movements in sports require the legs to move one at a time. Using lunges to improve the individual strength of the legs can help athletes run faster and jump higher. The lunge is an exercise to be incorporated in any athlete's training for any sport. Sports in which there is a lot of side stepping (volleyball, basketball, wrestling, or track and field) or sports in which athletes need to drive up on one leg can benefit from lunges.

Lunges are somewhat complex and require muscular strength, flexibility, and coordination in the lower body. Therefore, this exercise should not be done by beginners.

There are two basic variations to the lunge. First, and the one I like best for sports, is the walking lunge. The second is the step back lunge and is used when space is limited.

Lunges require very little equipment—an Olympic or standard bar placed on the back or dumbbells held to the side at arm's length. A squat or power rack can be used to rack the bar. If a rack is not available the athlete must pull the weight from the floor or use spotters to place the weight on the back. Walking lunges require a large open area with no obstructions. This can be in the weight room, a hallway, or a gym.

Spotting Technique

The lunge requires two spotters, one on each side of the bar. They will move along with the athlete as he or she does walking lunges. The role of the spotters is to grab the bar or assist the athlete if he or she is off balance.

Exercise Technique

The Walking Lunge

The athlete holds the weight strongly and securely up on the back. The body is erect with feet shoulder width apart (Figure 11.36a). Hands evenly spaced on the bar.

From this position the athlete takes a strong step forward with the dominant leg, usually the right leg (Figures 11.36b, 11.36c). The foot is planted heel first and rolled until the foot is flat on the floor (Figure 11.36d). The athlete should always make sure not to step to the side but straight forward, keeping the body in a straight line. From this position the athlete lowers the hips to the point where the top of the forward leg is *parallel* to the floor (Figure 11.36e). The knee does not move past the toes. The back leg is almost straight, its foot facing forward.

The hips should be lowered to knee level, centered under the body to prevent shifting to a side, and the upper body should be kept erect (athletes who have weak abdominals or poor flexibility will have a tendency to lean forward). The upper body is straight, chest out, head facing forward, and shoulders tight.

From this position, the athlete drives up with the front leg, pushes slightly forward with the back leg, and brings the body and weight up over the front leg. The upper body is kept straight at all times. The drive is forceful but under control. Now the athlete is in an erect position (Figure 11.36f). Then the athlete repeats the exercise with the opposite leg (Figures 11.36g, 11.36h, 11.36i, 11.36j, 11.36k). One repetition is the completion of a lunge with each leg. A set consists of several steps with each leg.

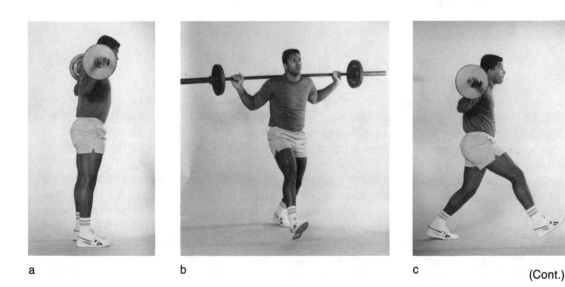

a   b   c   (Cont.)

Figure 11.36   Correct technique for the walking lunge.

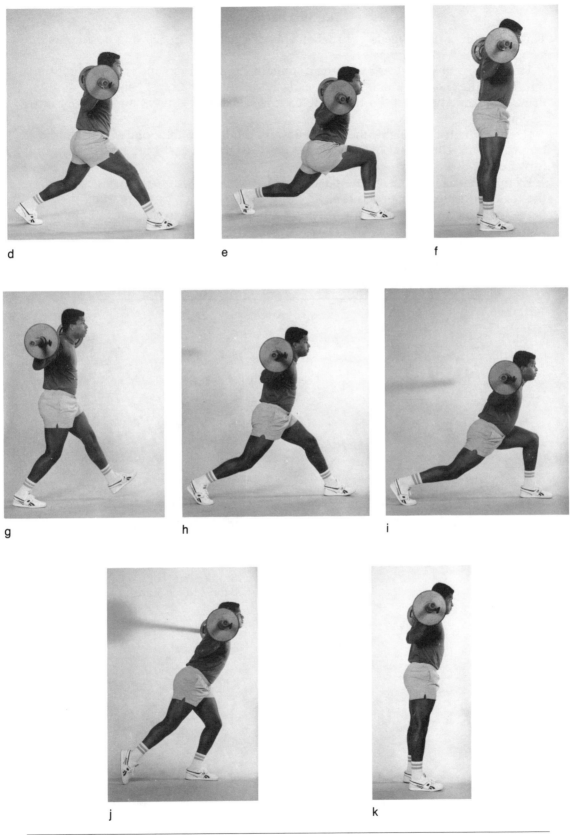

d   e   f

g   h   i

j   k

Figure 11.36   (Continued)

The Step Back Lunge

This variation of the lunge is used when space is limited. The starting position is the same as in the walking lunge.

The athlete moves forward with the dominant leg, heel first, and rolls the foot until it is flat on the floor. The athlete then bends at the knees and hips, being careful not to drive the front knee past the toes. The back leg is almost straight and the foot faces forward.

Keeping the back straight, the athlete lowers the hips to the point where the front thigh is parallel to the floor. The upper body is erect, chest out, and head facing forward.

From that position, the athlete pushes back forcefully with the forward leg, lifting the toes and pushing with the heel, to bring the body back to the starting position. Now, the athlete repeats with the other leg. Completing the exercise with both legs is one repetition.

COMMON ERRORS IN THE WALKING LUNGE

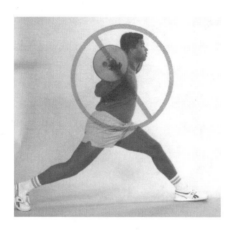

Figure 11.37   The athlete should not overstep.

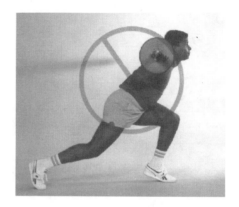

Figure 11.38   The weight should not be on the toes; the knees and body weight should not be pushed forward too much.

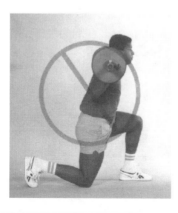

Figure 11.39   The back leg should not bend and touch the floor.

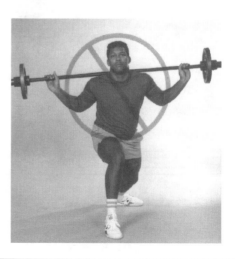

Figure 11.40   The back foot should not be pointing to the side.

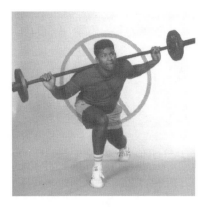

Figure 11.41   The body should not twist on the upward drive.

COACH'S CHECKLIST: WALKING LUNGE

☐ Bar loaded evenly, collars in place
☐ Bar placed high on upper back across traps and shoulders
☐ Hands comfortably holding bar
☐ Athlete stands straight, feet shoulder width apart
☐ Forward step with dominant leg, heel landing first
☐ Long but comfortable step
☐ Hips lowered until thigh parallel to floor
☐ Back leg remains straight
☐ Front foot flat on ground
☐ Front knee straight over toes
☐ Upper body kept upright
☐ Head up
☐ Chest up and out
☐ Momentary stop
☐ Push off with front leg up to standing position
☐ Movement under control
☐ Upper body stays erect
☐ Movement repeated with opposite leg

CHAPTER ● 12

Core Exercises for the Total Body

Complex total-body exercises require skill, joint stability, flexibility, and balance for athletes to perform them correctly. Therefore, they should be used to train athletes who are more advanced and have a solid background in strength training.

These exercises train athletes to work the total body against resistance in movements that more closely resemble the movements used in many sports. By training with these exercises you are improving the athlete's ability to generate force in similar patterns.

Because speed is a factor in these exercises (the bar must be moved quickly) the athlete's ability to generate power is improved. Study the formula for power (power = force × distance per unit time). With this formula you can demonstrate how total-body exercises help athletes improve their generation of power. The athlete is trained to move the weight quickly (to exert force) over the distance. By increasing the weight and/or speed the athlete is able to create more power and train the body to react explosively.

It will take more time for athletes to learn complex total-body exercises than simpler ones. You must be patient and teach exercises in steps by introducing only one portion of an exercise at a time and moving on to the next step only after the previous step is mastered. Some of the total-body exercises will need to be taught backwards, beginning with the last sequence and working toward the first sequence. Always begin with the easiest part and add the more complex parts as the athlete learns and progresses. This may take a few workouts, depending on the age and maturity of the athlete. Take your time; it is more important that the exercises be learned correctly, not speedily. When the athletes are taught in this way they will have a better chance of mastering the exercises and reducing the chance of injury. Done incorrectly, these exercises are of no benefit and can lead to injuries.

If you do not have the time, expertise, or facilities for athletes to perform these exercises, do not incorporate them into workouts.

It is necessary for athletes to see a total-body exercise performed in full by another athlete, either in the weight room or on video, before they begin. They need to see how the sequences work together and have a total picture of the properly executed exercise.

The visual image will help them create their own mental image before they attempt the steps leading to the total exercise.

Safety is foremost in the weight room, and the best way to obtain an atmosphere of safety is by teaching athletes the proper technique and the benefits of the exercise. The following safety guidelines apply to each of the following total-body exercises.

- Use proper lifting surface. Wood is probably the best. Never use a slippery surface such as concrete or tiles, nor a sticky surface such as carpet.
- Have a separate lifting area. A wooden platform is ideal, but a separate, marked-off area could be used. This is to keep other people from wandering into the area when someone is trying to concentrate and perform the exercise.
- Use the best bar in the house. The bar must be a straight Olympic bar with sleeves that rotate freely. A good bar minimizes elbow and wrist stress.
- Instruct athletes to wear shoes that have strong ankle support and a hard sole. Shoes that have these features prevent ankle and knee injuries. Running shoes are not recommended; tennis shoes or lifting shoes are the best.
- Use belts only as added support. Lifting belts help to stabilize the back and give abdominal support but do not prevent injuries.
- Allow wrist straps for particular situations. Wrist straps are useful when athletes are doing many repetitions. They help them hold on to the bar longer. Since you are trying to strengthen the body's major muscle groups, you do not want the grip to prevent athletes from completing all the sets and reps. An advanced athlete may want to use straps when doing few reps with a lot of weight.

  A beginner should not use straps. And straps should neither be used in warm-up sets, nor when the bar is pulled over the head.
- Use rubber bumper plates of different weight in the weight room. Bumper plates are useful. The lighter plates have the same diameter as heavier weights, and this enables the bar to be positioned at the right height off the floor whether you use lighter or heavier weights. Also, the bumper plates allow the bar to be dropped to the floor without any damage.
- Teach athletes how to push the bar away from their body and let it drop if the lift is not correct, if the athlete gets off balance, or if he or she is not able to rack the bar. The athlete should then step back from the bar and let it drop. It is always safer to let the bar drop than to try to save a bad lift and risk injury.

HIGH PULL

The high pull, the easiest of all explosive pulling exercises, is the core of all pulling movements. If the high pull is not mastered the athlete should not move on to the power clean or power snatch.

This total-body exercise works the legs, hips, lower back, upper back, and shoulders simultaneously. The calves and ankles are also worked when the athlete goes up on the toes. As the knees are extended the hamstrings and quadriceps are worked as well. Because of hip drive, the muscles of the lower back and the entire hip area are also strengthened. The upper back (lats and trapezius) are worked when the weight is shrugged and pulled up. The shoulders and biceps get some work when the athlete pulls with the arms, bringing the bar close to the chin.

The high pull is more than just a strength builder. It is performed quickly and explosively, training each of the working muscles to be more powerful. Since almost any sport in today's athletics requires hip movement and leg extension, the high pull becomes one of those exercises that benefit all sports. The muscle movement is very similar to jumping, throwing, running, and tackling. Its benefits can be seen in rebounding in basketball and in jumping at the volleyball net, to name two. The exercise develops power in the lower body, which translates directly into faster, more explosive athletes.

Exercise Technique

Breathing

The athlete inhales at the bottom in the pulling stance and holds the breath during the entire pull to the top. The athlete slowly exhales while lowering the bar to the starting position.

The Start

The athlete places his or her legs close to the bar, shins slightly touching the bar. The feet should be placed hip width apart, with the toes pointing slightly outward.

The athlete squats down, grabbing the bar with an overhand grip, slightly wider than shoulder width. The elbows should be turned out and the shoulders placed over the bar (Figure 12.1).

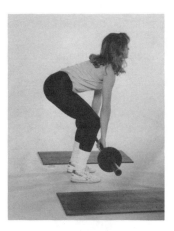

Figure 12.1   The start.

The athlete's body weight should be on the balls of the feet, with heels in contact with the ground.

Knees are placed inside the arms, with forearms slightly touching the thighs. In this position the athlete should be sitting back, with hips in line with the knees, thighs almost parallel to the floor. The back is at a 45-degree angle with the floor but held very straight.

The athlete should be looking forward in a relaxed position and should not tip his or her head all the way back in an attempt to keep the back straight. The shoulders should be squared with the chest out over the bar. The shoulders square with the chest because of the 45 degree angle of the back to the floor.

The First Pull

The athlete eases the bar off the floor, using legs and hips while keeping the back and arms straight. Hips and shoulders go up together at the same speed. The athlete should have the feeling of driving his or her legs through the floor. The bar is kept close to the shins and the feet are flat on the floor (Figure 12.2).

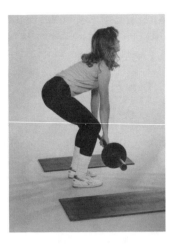

Figure 12.2   The pull.

The Second Pull

The bar should not be pulled around the knees, but the knees are pulled back so that the bar can come up in a straight line. The knees are pushed back by keeping the focus on driving the feet into the floor.

Just after the bar passes the knees they must be pushed back under the bar. This is where we get the stretch reflex, a critical point in the high pull (Figure 12.3).

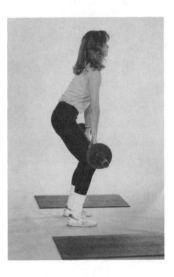

Figure 12.3   The power position.

It is important that the athlete pull the bar upward in a straight line, move the knees back until the bar has passed, then move back under the bar to get into the power or athlete position. In the power position the athlete's knees are bent, the body weight is still on the balls and heels of the feet, the back is straight and almost erect, and the head faces forward. The bar is hanging from the athlete's arms, which are still straight. This is where the athlete is the strongest. Now the athlete is able to exert maximum force, pulling the bar forcefully but in a controlled manner. This phase is commonly called the second pull.

At this point the athlete extends the legs and hips, driving up on the toes and shrugging the weight all the way up (Figure 12.4a). Make sure the athlete is going to raise the bar as much as possible by extending his or her knees and hips and by shrugging the shoulders all the way up to the ears (Figure 12.4b).

When the body has been fully extended, the bar has picked up momentum and *now* the bar can be pulled, using the arms and keeping the elbows out and high. The bar must be pulled using the total body (Figure 12.4c). To return the bar to the floor the athlete should lower the bar to the thighs and then to the floor by bending at the knees and hips.

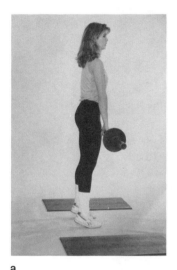
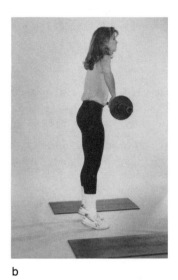
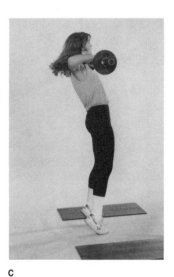

a   b   c

Figure 12.4   The second pull.

COMMON ERRORS IN THE HIGH PULL

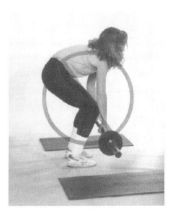
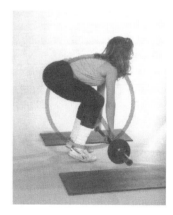

Figure 12.5   The back should not be rounded during the pull.

Figure 12.6   The athlete's weight should not be on the toes but on the entire foot.

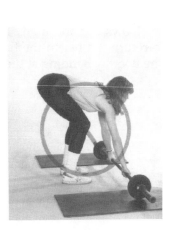

Figure 12.7 The bar should not be away from the body, nor should the hips be higher than the shoulders.

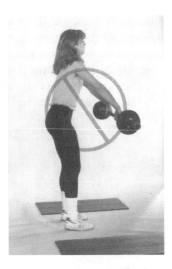

Figure 12.8 During the pull, do not pull the weight away from the body.

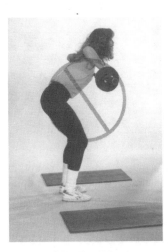

Figure 12.9 Do not dip down to the bar.

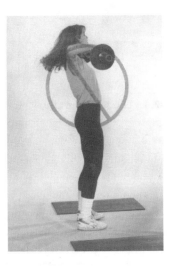

Figure 12.10 During the second pull, the athlete should not remain flat-footed or pull with just the arms.

COACH'S CHECKLIST: HIGH PULL

☐ Feet approximately shoulder width apart
☐ Toes pointing out slightly
☐ Feet flat on floor
☐ Bar touching shins
☐ Overhand grip, thumbs around bar
☐ Arms locked
☐ Back straight, face forward
☐ Thighs parallel to floor
☐ Shoulders back, chest out
☐ Chest over bar
☐ Bar eased off floor
☐ Bar comes up straight (not around knees)
☐ Bar stays close to body
☐ Bar passes knees
☐ Knees move back under bar
☐ Bar touches top of thighs
☐ Bar pulled explosively
☐ Body extended, athlete drives up on toes
☐ Bar pulled closed to body
☐ Traps shrugged to elevate bar
☐ Upward pull continued with arms
☐ Elbows kept high
☐ Bar lowered under control

POWER CLEAN

The power clean is sometimes misunderstood as a dangerous exercise. Those who have this opinion usually lack knowledge and understanding of the exercise. The power clean is not dangerous, but like any other exercise it can be dangerous if done incorrectly or with improper weight load. If you realize you cannot teach the exercise or are in a situation where the power clean cannot be done, then do not incorporate it into the program.

In this total-body exercise the athlete is training the legs, hips, lower back, upper back, and shoulders (similar to the high pull). The calves and ankles are worked when the athletes go up on their toes; when they extend their knees, the hamstrings and quadriceps are worked. Because of hip rotation, the muscles of the lower back and the entire hip area (gluteus maximus and hip muscles) are also strengthened. The upper back (lats and trapezius) are worked when the weight is pulled up in shrugging. The shoulders and biceps get some work when the bar is pulled with the arms. There is even some shoulder girdle development when the bar is racked and the elbows brought forward.

This exercise is beneficial to all sports that require quick bursts—track, football, basketball, and wrestling, to name a few. Like the high pull, the power clean is done quickly and explosively. It has been proven that pulling movements, such as those in the power clean, produce maximum human power during the execution.

Exercise Technique

Breathing

The athlete inhales at the bottom when in the pulling stance and holds the breath during the entire pull to the top. The athlete slowly exhales while lowering the bar to the starting position

The Start

The beginning of the power clean is the same as in the high pull. The athlete approaches the bar and places the legs close to the bar, shins slightly touching the bar. The feet should be placed hip width apart, with the toes pointing slightly outward.

The athlete squats down, grabbing the bar with an overhand grip, slightly wider than shoulder width. The elbows should be turned out and the shoulders placed over the bar. The body weight should be on the balls of the feet, with heels in contact with the floor. The knees are placed inside the arms, with forearms slightly touching the thighs (Figure 12.11a). The athlete should be sitting back, hips in line with the knees, thighs almost parallel to the floor.

The back is at as 45-degree angle with the floor but held very straight. The shoulders should be squared with the chest out over the bar (Figure 12.11b).

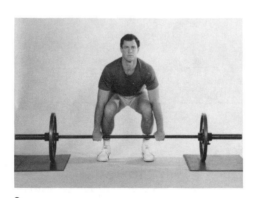

a

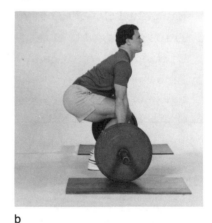

b

Figure 12.11   The start.

The First Pull

The athlete eases the bar off the floor, using the legs and hips while keeping the back flat. The arms are kept straight throughout the pull. The athlete should have the feeling of driving his or her legs through the floor. The bar is kept close to the shins, and feet are flat on the floor (Figure 12.12a, b).

The bar is not to be pulled around the knees, but the knees are pushed back so the bar can come up in a straight line (Figure 12.12c). Just after the bar passes the knees they must be pushed back under the bar (Figure 12.12d, e). This is the power position, a critical point in the power clean. Here the athlete's knees are bent, the body weight is still on the balls and heels of the feet, and the bar is hanging from the arms (Figure 12.12f).

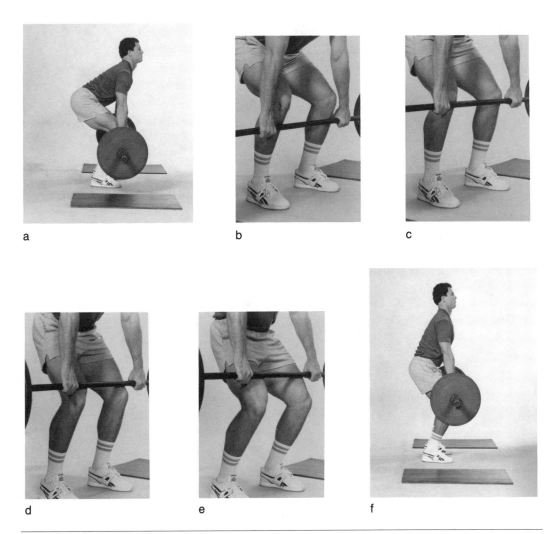

a   b   c

d   e   f

Figure 12.12   The first pull.

The Second Pull

At this point the athlete extends the legs, goes up on the toes, and shrugs the weight all the way up (Figure 12.13a, b).

After fully extending the body, the athlete can pull the bar with his or her arms, keeping the elbows out and high (Figure 12.13c, d). The bar has to be pulled very high, and when it reaches the highest point the athlete moves under the bar by bending at the knees and spreading the feet slightly to the side (Figure 12.13e). The weight is racked evenly across the shoulders, elbows are high, back is straight, and head is up. When the bar is securely racked the athlete stands up.

The athlete should lower the bar to the thighs and then to the floor by bending at the knees and hips.

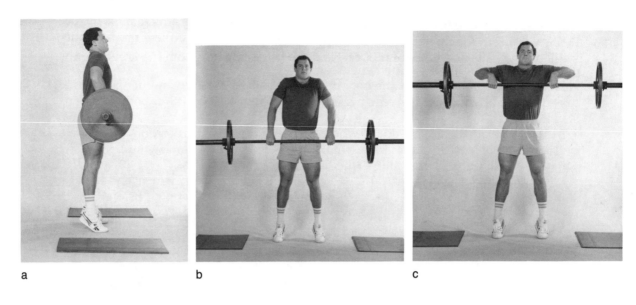

a   b   c

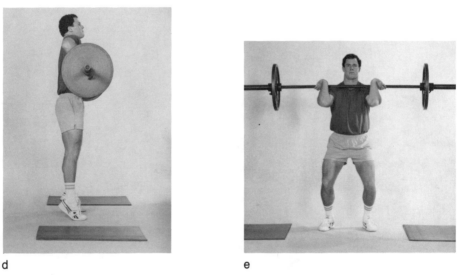

d   e

Figure 12.13   The second pull.

Teaching the Power Clean

When teaching a complex exercise such as the power clean, break the exercise down into its different parts and start with the easiest, adding the more complex movements as you go along.

Step 1 in teaching the power clean is to teach the athlete to stand straight and hold the bar while doing a shrug. This means lifting the bar just by shrugging the shoulders as high as possible toward the ears, while always keeping the arms straight.

In step 2 the athlete bends slightly at the knees and hips, then pulls the weight up by extending them, going up on the toes and shrugging the shoulders as in step 1. This is often called the power shrug. In this movement the athlete achieves total lower-body extension.

Step 3 is the same as step 2, but after the body is extended and the shoulders are shrugged, the athlete pulls the bar to the chest, using the arms. The bar is kept very close to the body during the entire movement. This phase is called the power pull.

Step 4 begins at the power position, with legs slightly bent. The athlete pulls the bar up, as in step 3, but when the bar reaches its highest point the athlete moves under the bar by bending the knees and racking the bar onto the shoulders, pointing the elbows out and high. This is the hang clean.

Notice that up to this point the only difference from one step to another is that one movement is added. The bar remains close to the body and all other body positions stay the same.

In step 5 the athlete tries to do the whole exercise from the floor position. The athlete pulls the weight past the knees to the thighs, stops momentarily, makes sure he or she is in good position, and does step 4, the hang clean.

When the athlete has mastered the exercise in this step-by-step manner, the exercise should be repeated frequently in the power position without stopping between each step.

COMMON ERRORS IN THE POWER CLEAN

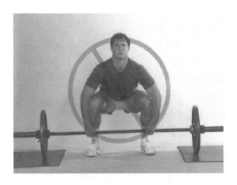

Figure 12.14 Athletes might have a tendency to start the exercise with the arms bent and legs too far apart.

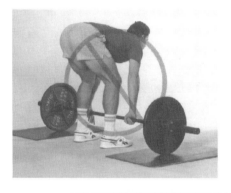

Figure 12.15 The hips should not be higher than the shoulders.

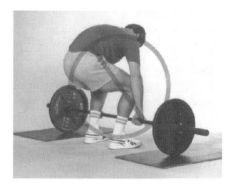

Figure 12.16 The back should not be rounded and head facing down.

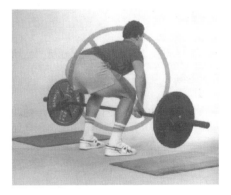

Figure 12.17 The athlete should not jerk the bar off the floor by pulling with the arms first.

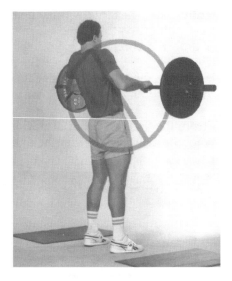

Figure 12.18 The weight should not be muscled up by using only the arms.

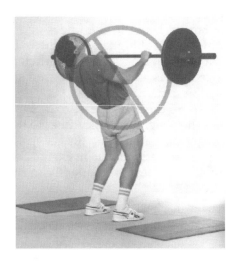

Figure 12.19 At the end of the pull, the athlete should not lean back and swing the bar upward.

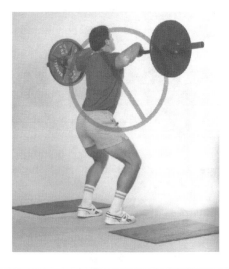

Figure 12.20 The athlete should not dip down toward the bar but should pull the bar as high as possible.

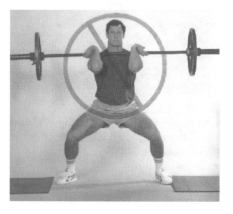

Figure 12.21 When racking the bar on the shoulders, the athlete should not spread the feet too far apart.

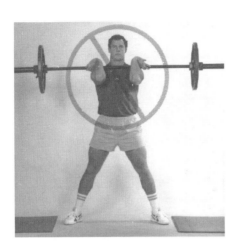

Figure 12.22 When racking the bar, the athlete should not keep the legs straight.

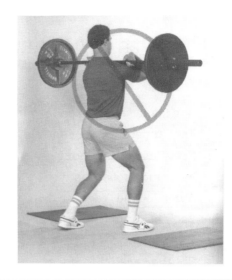

Figure 12.23 The athlete should not step back when racking the bar onto the shoulders.

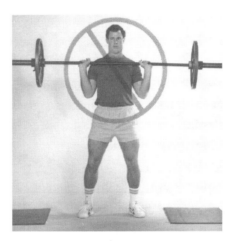

Figure 12.24 When supporting the bar on the shoulders, the athlete should not point the elbows down.

COACH'S CHECKLIST: POWER CLEAN

- ☐ Bar loaded evenly, collars in place
- ☐ Feet approximately shoulder width apart
- ☐ Feet flat on the floor
- ☐ Bar touching shins
- ☐ Arms locked, regular grip, thumbs around bar
- ☐ Back straight
- ☐ Head facing forward
- ☐ Thighs parallel to floor
- ☐ Shoulders over bar
- ☐ Easy pull off floor
- ☐ Bar comes up straight (not around knees)
- ☐ Knees move back
- ☐ Bar stays close to body
- ☐ Bar passes knees
- ☐ Knees move back under bar
- ☐ Bar touching top of thighs
- ☐ Back tight, arms straight
- ☐ Body extends fully, athlete up on toes
- ☐ Traps are shrugged to elevate bar
- ☐ Continued upward pull by pulling with arms
- ☐ Weight racked across top of shoulders
- ☐ Elbows point out and high
- ☐ Feet spread slightly to side
- ☐ Athlete stands up, under control
- ☐ Bar lowered under control to top of thighs
- ☐ Bar lowered to floor, athlete bends at knees and hips

POWER SNATCH

The power snatch is a super exercise for developing total-body strength, particularly in the legs, hips, back, and shoulders. This exercise and the power clean have many similarities. Both are time-saving multijoint exercises and have the same benefits in hip rotation and development of power. The power snatch strengthens the same muscles as the power clean, but because the weight must be pulled high over the head there is additional development of the upper back and shoulders.

The purpose of the exercise is to move the weight quickly and explosively in one good pull. Because of the long pull required in doing a power snatch (i.e., pulling the weight all the way from the floor to above the head) the athlete will use a lot less weight than in any other pulling exercise.

This exercise is quite advanced and should not be performed by beginning or intermediate athletes. It is the fourth pulling exercise an athlete learns. The athlete must be able to do the dead lift, the high pull, and the power clean correctly before attempting the power snatch.

When learning the exercise, the athlete should start with a broomstick and move up to an empty bar. The weight should increase progressively as the athlete matures and masters the exercise. The technique is mastered in the same way as the power clean, by doing the last part of the exercise first and working toward the beginning.

Exercise Technique

Breathing

The athlete inhales at the bottom when in the pulling stance and holds the breath during the entire pull to the top. The athlete slowly exhales while lowering the bar to the starting position.

The Grip and Stance

The athlete should use a wide grip, each hand 6 to 10 inches from the bar sleeve. Feet should be flat on the floor, approximately 12 inches (hip width) apart, with the body weight evenly distributed over the feet and toes pointing out slightly. The shins should be slightly touching the bar. Hips should be low and thighs nearly parallel to the floor and at an angle to the shins between 90 and 100 degrees (Figure 12.25a). The back should be straight and at angle of about 45 degrees with the floor. These favorable angles assure a strong position for getting the bar off the floor.

With the head up, in line with the spine and facing forward, the athlete should place his or her shoulders over the bar and force the shoulder blades together and chest out. Arms should be straight and the whole body tight and powerful in an isometric contraction (Figure 12.25b).

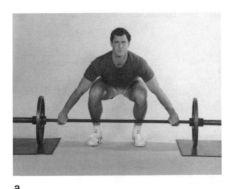
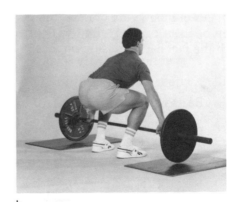

a   b

Figure 12.25 Correct grip and stance.

The First Pull

The athlete should pull the bar off the floor slowly (no jerky movements) by pushing with the legs and raising the hips. The athlete should have the feeling of pushing the feet straight through the floor. Arms remain straight throughout the movement (Figure 12.26a).

The pull from this point up to the knees should be gradual. Keeping the bar close to the knees, the athlete extends the legs and moves the knees back to make room for the bar to pass straight up (the bar does not move around the knees). When the bar has passed the knees, they are moved back under the bar, creating the power position (Figure 12.26b).

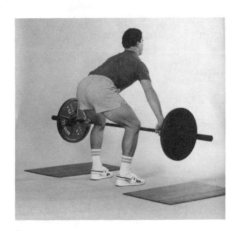
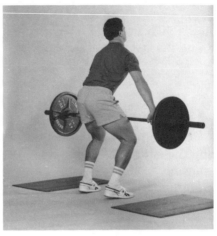

a   b

Figure 12.26   The first pull.

The Second Pull

From the power position the athlete can exert maximum power and pull the bar up forcefully and high by extending the hips and legs fully, going up on the toes, and shrugging the shoulders as high as possible (Figure 12.27a).

At this time the athlete bends the arms and continues the upward pull of the bar. The body is kept upright and should not lean back (Figure 12.27b); the bar should be kept close. Elbows are out and the bar is pulled as high as possible. The athlete should keep heels in contact with the floor as long as possible to continue the upward drive with the feet before raising on toes.

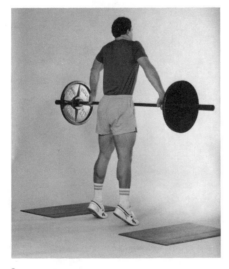
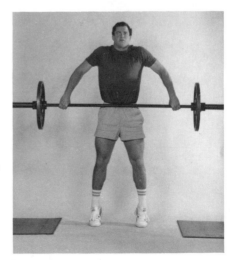

a   b

Figure 12.27   The second pull.

Over the Top

Once the bar has reached its maximum height, the athlete spreads the feet slightly to the side, bends at the knees, and pulls the weight overhead (Figure 12.28a). In this movement the wrists should turn so the bar rotates. This last phase is a very quick, strong movement that brings the bar overhead with straight arms. The arms should not bend while bringing the bar overhead, then straighten.

When the bar is secured over the head, the athlete extends the legs (Figure 12.28b). From this finished position the athlete slowly lowers the bar down to the thighs and then to the floor by bending at the knees and hips.

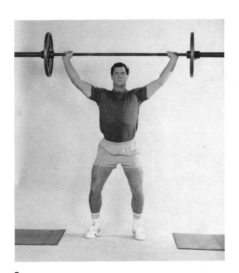
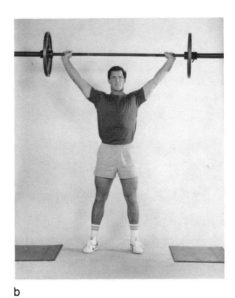

a

b

Figure 12.28   Over the top.

COMMON ERRORS IN THE POWER SNATCH

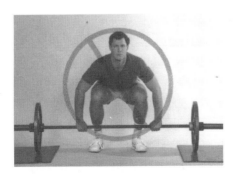
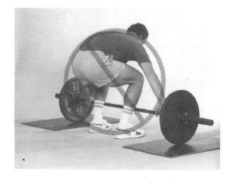

Figure 12.29   Hand placement should not be close as in the power clean but wide and close to the end of the bar.

Figure 12.30   The back should not be rounded during the exercise.

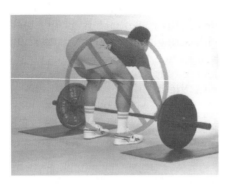

Figure 12.31   The hips should not be too high or the bar away from the body.

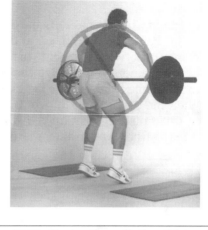

Figure 12.32   During the pull, the athlete should not pull with the arms before extending the body.

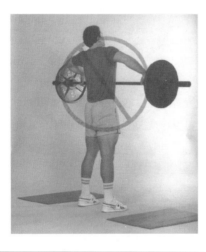

Figure 12.33   The athlete should not muscle the bar up by keeping the feet flat and pulling just with the arms.

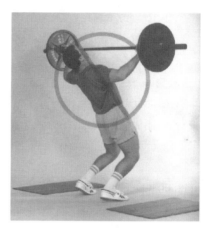

Figure 12.34   The athlete should not swing the bar out and up while bending the body backward.

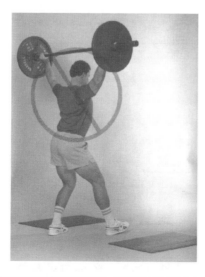

Figure 12.35   The athlete should not step back in the recovery phase.

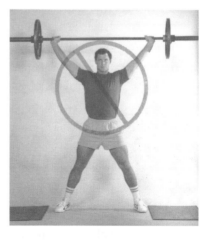

Figure 12.36   The legs should not be kept straight during the recovery phase.

COACH'S CHECKLIST: POWER SNATCH

☐ Hands placed close to end of bar
☐ Feet flat, shoulder width apart, toes slightly out
☐ Bar touching shins
☐ Arms straight
☐ Chest up and out, shoulder blades together
☐ Head facing forward
☐ Back straight
☐ Hips low with thighs parallel to floor
☐ Bar pulled slowly off floor in a straight line
☐ Arms straight
☐ Pull done with legs and hips
☐ Knees move back and return under the bar
☐ Back straight
☐ Athlete bends at hips
☐ Arms straight
☐ Bar slightly over knees and touching thighs
☐ Legs and hips extend
☐ Shoulder shrug
☐ Pull with arms
☐ Bar remains close to body
☐ Legs spread slightly to side
☐ Athlete bends at hips and knees
☐ Bar pulled over the head
☐ Body extended, bar held high overhead

CHAPTER
13

Auxiliary Exercises

All workouts need to be supplemented with a variety of auxiliary exercises. The combination of core and auxiliary exercises will ensure that all muscle areas are strength trained. Auxiliary exercises can be used to isolate and strengthen specific areas and can provide sport-specific strength training. Some auxiliary exercises may be more important than others, depending on the sport and specific skills of the athlete. Because neck strength is very important to football players and wrestlers, they will do neck exercises extensively, whereas tennis or golf athletes will not.

The following exercises are very simple. They are easily implemented with basic equipment and are applicable to all sports. The larger the variety of equipment you have, the more variations are possible.

NECK EXERCISES

A strong neck is necessary to help reduce the chance of neck injury in sports where contact is made with the upper body. The power clean, high pulls, and shrug movements work the trapezius muscle, which is important in strengthening the neck. But the neck also needs to be strengthened in its four moving planes. The first plane, neck flexion, moves the head forward toward the chest. The second, neck extension, pushes the head back toward the shoulders. The third, right lateral flexion, moves the right ear toward the right shoulder. The fourth, left lateral flexion, moves the left ear toward the left shoulder.

Manual Resistance Exercises

When no machines are available, a partner can apply the resistance. It is critical that the partner know the trainee well and understand how much resistance is needed. The partners need to communicate and work together for better results.

The athlete lies securely on a bench, head hanging off the end of the bench. The partner stands near the athlete and, using a towel for comfort and stability, adds resistance. To warm up the muscles, very little resistance is applied in the first few reps.

The resistance is gradual and constant, increasing as the repetitions progress. Each repetition takes 4 or 5 seconds to execute the full range of motion, stopping momentarily when the action is finished, then returning to the starting position. For neck flexion the partner places resistance in the forehead area, and the athlete pushes up toward the chest (Figures 13.1a, b, c, d). For neck extension the partner puts pressure on the back of the athlete's head, and the athlete pushes upward toward the shoulders (Figures 13.2a, b, c). For right lateral flexion, pressure is put on the right side of the head, which the athlete pushes toward the right shoulder (Figures 13.3a, b). For left lateral flexion the partner places resistance on the left side of the head, and the athlete pushes toward the left shoulder (Figure 13.4a, b, c). One rep consists of completing the exercise on all four sides.

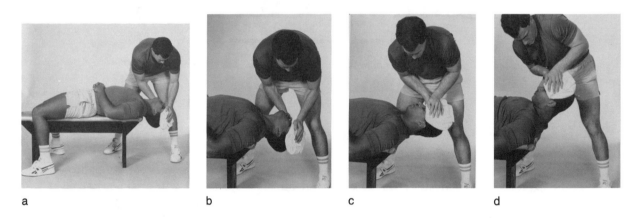

a b c d

Figure 13.1 Neck flexion with manual resistance.

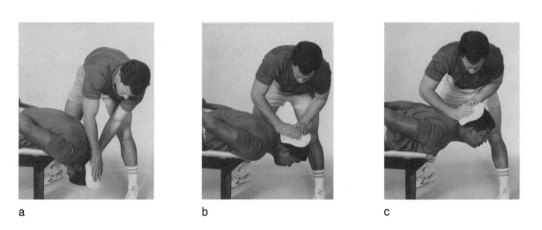

a b c

Figure 13.2 Neck extension with manual resistance.

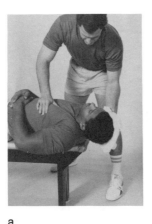
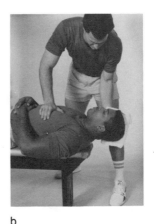

a   b

Figure 13.3   Right lateral flexion with manual resistance.

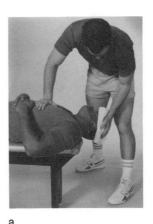
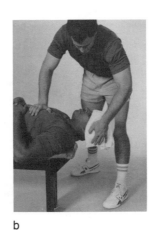
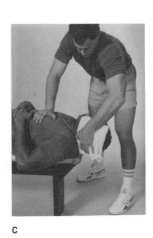

a   b   c

Figure 13.4   Left lateral flexion with manual resistance.

Variable Resistance Machines Exercises

All neck strengthening machines do basically the same thing. Sitting comfortably, the athlete grabs the handles for torso stability (Figure 13.5). The head pads should be placed so there is free movement in a full range of motion. During the exercise the torso and shoulders do not move. All movement is done with the head. Forcing, jamming, or explosive movements are forbidden. Movements must be done slowly and under control. The athlete exerts force against the pad in a full range of motion on all four sides (front, back, right side, left side) (Figures 13.6a-h).

SHOULDER EXERCISES

Shoulder exercises work primarily the deltoid muscles. The deltoids are a group of three specific muscles: the anterior, middle, and posterior deltoids. To train properly all parts of the shoulder, resistance must be moved in different planes.

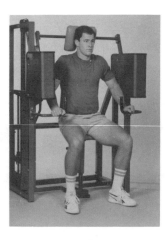

Figure 13.5   Starting position on the neck machine.

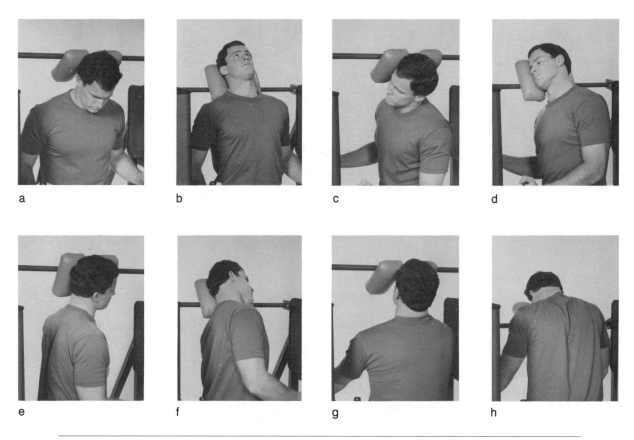

Figure 13.6   Range of motion on the neck machine.

Alternate Incline Dumbbell Presses

To support the athlete's back and to allow more weight to be used, the athlete sits on an incline utility bench with an angle of 45 degrees or more. The athlete's back and head are resting on the bench, with legs to the side and feet flat on the floor. The athlete takes a dumbbell in each hand, resting them close to the shoulders. Elbows should be out and to the side in line with the shoulders (Figure 13.7a).

Keeping the left dumbbell down the athlete pushes the right dumbbell up in complete extension straight over the face (Figure 13.7b). The dumbbell is held momentarily in this position, then brought down slowly (Figure 13.7c). The athlete completes the same movement with the left dumbbell (Figure 13.7d, e). Both sides completed equals one rep.

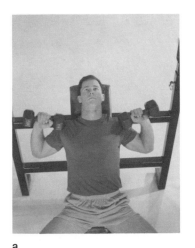
a

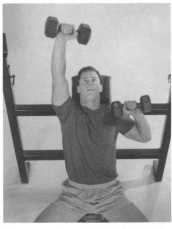
b

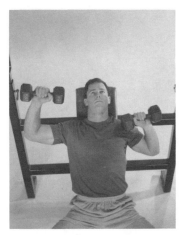
c

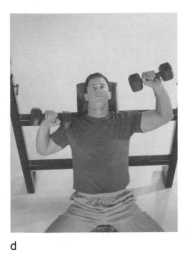
d

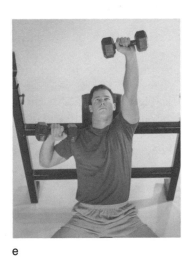
e

Figure 13.7   Alternate incline dumbbell presses.

Shoulders and head should not be lifted off the bench. The dumbbells should be brought all the way down to the shoulder for full range of motion. The athlete should never use momentum to bring the dumbbell up (i.e., bouncing at the bottom). The shoulders should be doing the work. As a variation the athlete may push both dumbbells up and down at the same time.

Dumbbell Lateral Raises

The athlete stands with feet shoulder width apart, body straight, and head facing forward. While holding the palms inward, the athlete holds the dumbbells (weights) in front (Figure 13.8a). The athlete then raises the dumbbells sideways (Figure 13.8b) to a position basically parallel to the floor, stops momentarily (Figure 13.8c), then slowly lowers to the starting position.

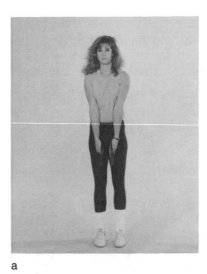
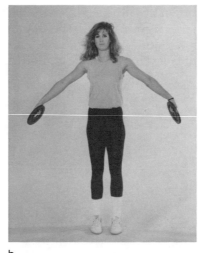
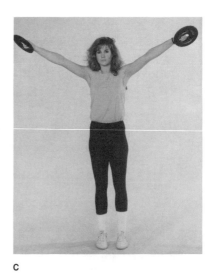

a   b   c

Figure 13.8   Dumbbell lateral raises.

Be sure the athlete keeps the dumbbells in line with the shoulders. Some athletes may have a tendency to drive their elbows forward. The athlete should never sling the dumbbells up to gain momentum. The body is kept still. Each repetition begins from a dead stop. The dumbbells should not be twisted at the top of the movement.

Dumbbell Front Raises

The athlete stands with feet shoulder width apart, body straight, and head facing forward. Arms are to the side, and the athlete holds the dumbbells with the palms facing back (Figure 13.9a). The dumbbells are raised forward, the forearms rising to a position basically parallel to the floor (Figure 13.9b). This position is held momentarily (Figure 13.9c), then the athlete slowly lowers the dumbbells to the starting position. The body keeps still, allowing the shoulders to do all the work.

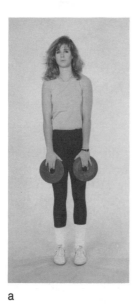
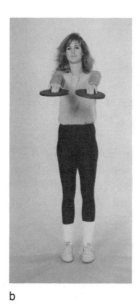
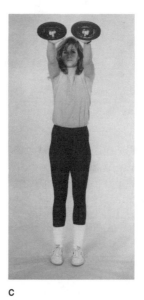

a   b   c

Figure 13.9   Dumbbell front raises.

Bent Over Rear Dumbbell Raises

Standing with feet shoulder width apart, the athlete bends at the hips so the torso is almost parallel to the floor. The athlete holds a strong position, chest out, shoulders back, head up, and facing forward. The dumbbells are held down with palms facing each other (Figure 13.10a). With the elbows kept slightly bent the dumbbells are raised up to the side (Figure 13.10b) until the forearms are in a position parallel to the floor. The parallel position is held momentarily (Figure 13.10c), then the athlete slowly lowers the dumbbells to the starting position. The athlete's hands should not turn inward. The movement is done vigorously but with no jerking or moving of the torso.

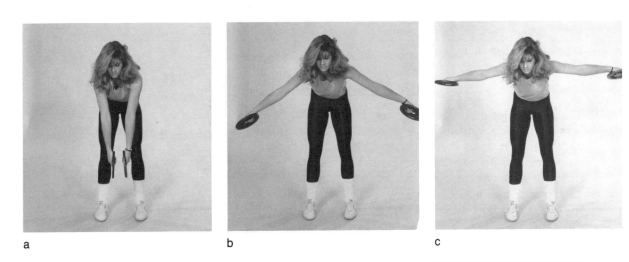

a   b   c

Figure 13.10   Bent-over rear dumbbell raises.

CHEST EXERCISES

For maximum development of the chest, workouts can be supplemented with very specific chest exercises. Athletes take a lot of pride in the development of their chest and often view a developed chest as an indication of strength.

Dumbbell Flies

The athlete lies on a flat utility bench, head resting on the bench, legs to the side, and feet flat on the floor. The palms are facing each other and the dumbbells are extended overhead (Figure 13.11a). Bending the elbows slightly, the athlete lowers the dumbbells in line with the shoulders, keeping the elbows pointed down and back (Figure 13.11b, c). The biggest mistake the athlete can make here is twisting the elbows. The shoulders, elbows, and dumbbells should form a straight line in the up-and-down movement. The athlete should lower the dumbbells as far as flexibility permits. A narrow bench provides greater range of motion in the shoulder area. At the bottom the athlete stops momentarily, then slowly brings the dumbbells back up to the starting position. At the top the dumbbells are touched together slightly. The head or shoulders should never come off the bench. The athlete should concentrate on contracting the chest muscles when pulling the dumbbells upward.

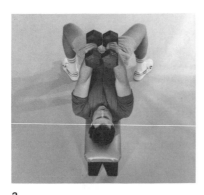
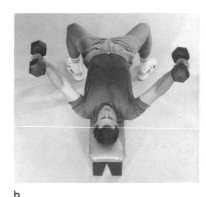
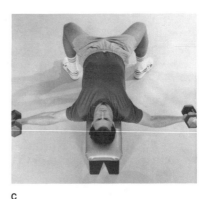

a   b   c

Figure 13.11   Dumbbell fly.

Straight-Arm Dumbbell Pullovers

The athlete lies on a flat utility bench with head hanging over the edge of the bench, legs to the side, and feet flat on the floor. The athlete holds one dumbbell with both hands and extends the arms over the chest (Figure 13.12a). Arms are held almost straight but with a very slight bend at the elbows. Keeping the arms in this position, the athlete moves the dumbbell in an arc behind the head and toward the floor (Figure 13.12b, c). It should be lowered as far as flexibility permits. At the bottom position the athlete pauses momentarily, then slowly brings the dumbbell back to the starting position. The work should be done by the chest muscles, not the hands.

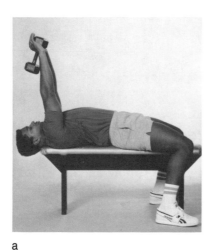
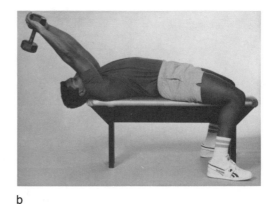

a   b

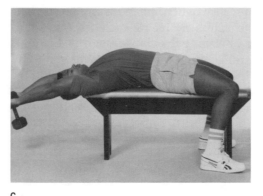

c

Figure 13.12   Straight-arm dumbbell pullovers.

ARM EXERCISES

Most athletes dream of having big arms, big triceps, and big biceps. Many athletes, however, neglect an important part of arm strength—wrist strength. Hand and forearm strength are especially important in sports where hands are used extensively (tennis, wrestling, football, baseball). Even though the arms may not be a major area in sport performance, arm workouts are important for total-body strength.

Bicep Curls

Standing with feet shoulder width apart and body erect, the athlete grabs the bar (straight or curl) about shoulder width apart and palms up. The bar rests in front, close to the legs, and the athlete's arms are straight (Figure 13.13a). The athlete curls the bar upward all the way to the chin, with elbows held close in (Figure 13b, c). The athlete stops momentarily at the top position, then slowly lowers the bar back to the starting position. There should be no hip or back movement. This exercise can also be done with dumbbells.

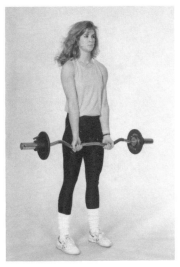
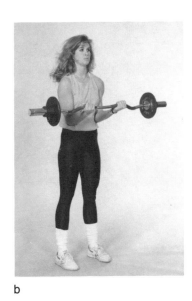
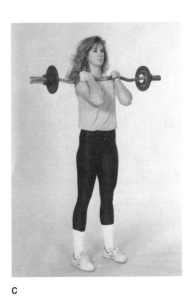

a   b   c

Figure 13.13   Bicep curls.

Tricep Extensions

The athlete lies on a bench, feet to the side, and hands slightly less than shoulder width apart. The athlete raises the bar to arm's length straight over the face (Figure 13.14a). By bending the elbows, the athlete slowly lowers the bar toward the forehead (Figure 13.14b). The upper arms are held close to the head, and the elbows are held close together. The bar is lowered to 90 degrees, stopped momentarily (Figure 13.14c), then brought back to starting position. The athlete should not bounce the bar at the bottom or open elbows out to the side in the upward movement.

Dips

Keeping the body straight and arms locked, the athletes use their arm muscles to lift their bodies (Figure 13.15a). The grip should be comfortable, slightly wider than shoulder width apart. For more comfort the knees can be bent and the right foot crossed over the left. The body lowers to the point where the upper arm is parallel to the floor (Figure 13.15b, c). The athletes stop momentarily then raise back up to the starting

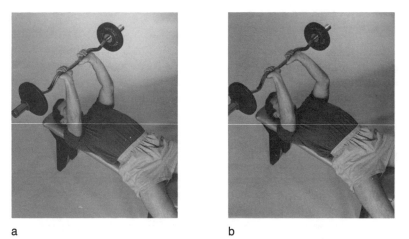
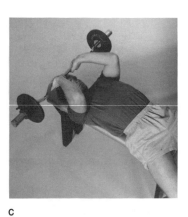

a   b   c

Figure 13.14   Tricep extensions.

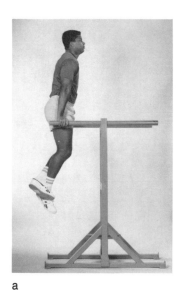
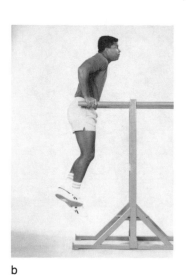
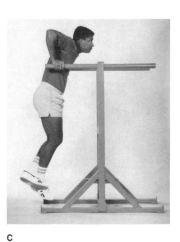

a   b   c

Figure 13.15   Dips.

position (arms fully extended). At the top the athletes stop momentarily and repeat the movement. During the upward drive the body should not swing or twist. All the work should be done by the triceps and shoulders.

To add resistance, weight can be tied around the athletes' waist with a special belt. Although this exercise is great for training triceps it also works the shoulders. If you do not wish to train the shoulders you should choose another tricep exercise.

Wrist Curls

The athlete kneels at the side of a flat utility bench and grabs the bar with hands about six inches apart. The forearms and elbows are placed flat on the bench for support and stability. The hands and bar will be hanging off the side of the bench for free movement and full range of motion (Figure 13.16a). When the palms are down the extensor muscles of the forearms are worked, and when the palms are up the wrist flexor muscles are worked. The athlete pulls the bar up as far as possible, using only the wrists (Figure

13.16b, c), stops momentarily, and slowly lowers the bar back to the starting position. At the bottom position the bar can be allowed to roll to the tips of the fingers for more wrist flexion. The athlete should roll it back into the hand before the next upward pull.

The exercise should be performed at a moderate speed, under control. A full range of motion can be from 100 to 160 degrees, depending on the athlete's wrist flexibility. If the weight is too heavy the athlete will not be able to perform the exercise in a full range of motion.

This exercise can also be performed seated, with the forearms resting on the quads, and it can be done with dumbbells.

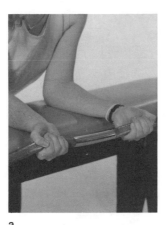
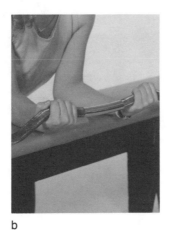
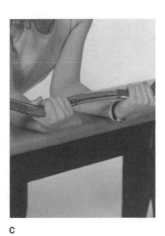

a   b   c

Figure 13.16 Wrist curls.

UPPER-BACK EXERCISES

Most athletes are more interested in developing the front part of the upper body—the chest—and will neglect its counterpart, the upper back. This is a very large, strong area that includes the trapezius, rhomboids, and latissimus dorsi as its main muscle groups. Upper-back strength is important in sports that require pulling movements (football, wrestling, swimming, and gymnastics, for example). Athletes in these sports will often have superior upper-back strength compared to other athletes.

Bent Over Rows

The athlete stands with feet shoulder width apart and grabs the bar with palms down, shoulder width apart (Figure 13.17a). The athlete bends at the knees and lowers the hips while bending the upper back forward to an almost parallel position to the floor. Shoulders are back (Figure 13.17b, c). The head is up, looking forward, and the torso is kept tight. The athlete slowly pulls the weight to the lower part of the chest, keeping the elbows out (Figure 13.17d). Then the athlete stops momentarily and lowers the bar slowly to the starting position. The athlete should never jerk the bar, lean toward the bar, or round the back.

Shoulder Shrugs

The athlete stands erect, with feet shoulder width apart, and holds the bar close to the body with straight arms, palms down, and hands about shoulder width apart (Figure 13.18a). The athlete raises the weight by shrugging the shoulders toward the ears. There should be no pulling movement with the arms. All the work should be done

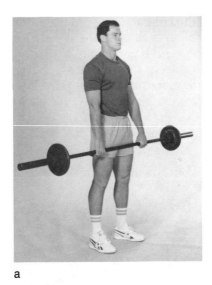
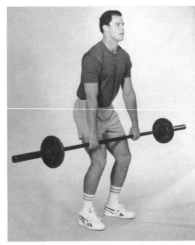
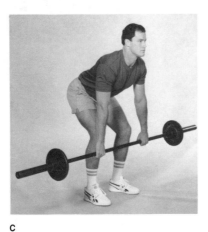
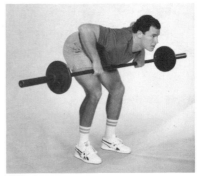

Figure 13.17 Bent-over rows.

with traps. The head is kept still while the shoulders are elevated as high as possible in a straight upward line (Figure 13.18b, c). The shoulders should not rotate. The athlete momentarily holds the weight at the top, then slowly lowers it back to the starting position.

Pull-Ups

The athlete grabs the bar wider than shoulder width apart, with palms down and thumbs around the bar (Figure 13.19a). The wider the grip the more the lats are used in the pulling movement. The athlete hangs from the bar with arms extended, legs bent, and feet crossed. The athlete pulls up until the pull-up bar touches the back of the neck, pauses momentarily, then lowers gradually to the starting position (Figure 13.19b, c). The body should not twist or swing in this exercise.

Upright Rows

The athlete stands with feet shoulder width apart and hands placed on the bar 8 to 10 inches apart, with palms facing down (Figure 13.20a). The arms are straight, and the athlete holds the bar close to the body at arm's length. The bar is pulled upward in a

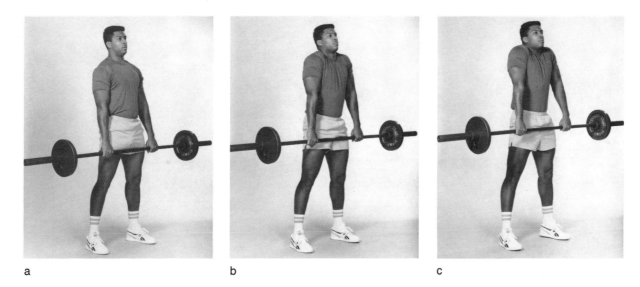

Figure 13.18 Shoulder shrugs.

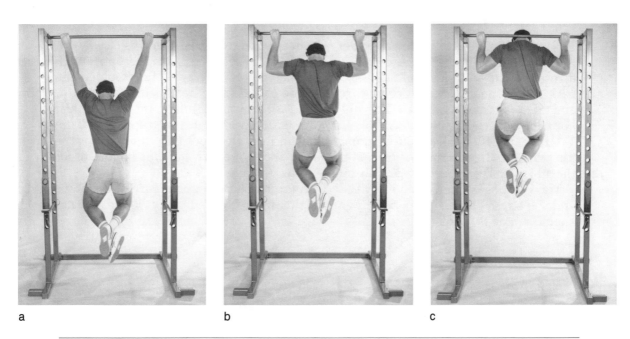

Figure 13.19 Pull-ups.

straight line to the chin (Figure 13.20b, c). During the movement the elbows are kept high and held beside the head. At the top the athlete stops momentarily then lowers the bar to the starting position. This action should be done slowly with no swinging or jerking to create momentum. The legs are kept straight throughout the exercise, and the athlete should not lean back at the top of the lift. The arms should be completely extended before the athlete begins the next repetition.

LOWER-BACK EXERCISES

Only some core exercises—dead lifts, power cleans, high pulls, power snatches—will train the lower back, and often this area is overlooked and untrained. The main muscles worked in the lower back are the spinal erectors.

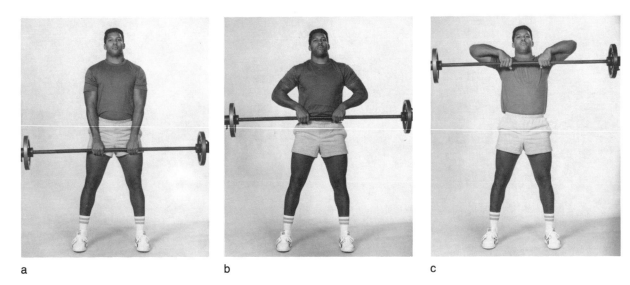

a   b   c

Figure 13.20   Upright rows.

Good Mornings

The athlete stands with feet shoulder width apart and hands evenly spaced with thumbs around the bar (Figure 13.21a). The bar is racked evenly on the upper back across the traps, but it should not be racked too high on the traps. The shoulders are back so the shoulder blades come together. The chest is out, head is facing forward, and the torso has a slight arch. The athlete bends slightly at the knees, then at the hips. Hips move back slightly as the torso is lowered almost parallel to the floor (Figure 13.21b, c, d). The athlete pauses momentarily at the bottom position, then moves the torso back to the starting position. Hips extend and move forward. It is important for the athlete to keep the torso tight throughout the movement.

This exercise is often done incorrectly with too much weight. Because of the angle and the stress on the lower back, light weights must be used. Very young athletes should not do this exercise.

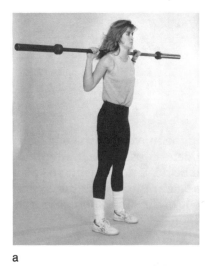

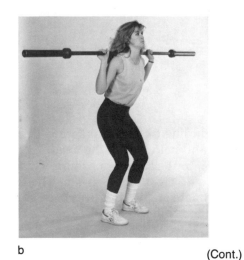

a   b   (Cont.)

Figure 13.21   Good mornings.

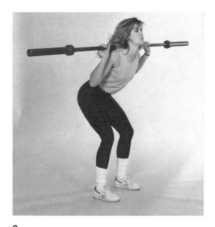
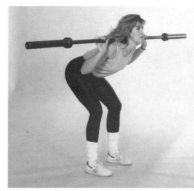

c

d

Figure 13.21   (Continued)

Back Raises

Back raises can be performed using specific equipment or a flat utility bench and a training partner. The training partner will hold the athlete's legs down.

The athlete lies prone on the apparatus. The pad should be under the thighs to permit free movement of the hips and lower back. The feet are securely supported under the foot holders and the torso hangs over the end of the apparatus. The back is straight, shoulders back, chest out, and head in line with the torso. The arms are crossed on the chest or behind the head for added resistance (Figure 13.22a). The athlete bends at the hips and lowers the torso until it is perpendicular to the floor, maintaining a tight, strong upper and lower back (Figure 13.22b, c, d). The athlete stops momentarily and, using lower-back muscles, slowly raises the torso back to the starting position. The athlete should not hyperextend, twist, or bounce at the bottom to gain momentum. The exercise is performed at moderate speed under control.

For the more advanced athlete with good lower-back strength, a weight plate can be held for added resistance.

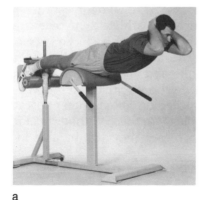
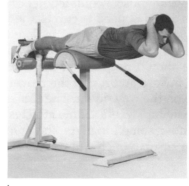

a

b

(Cont.)

Figure 13.22   Back raises.

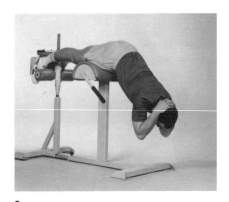
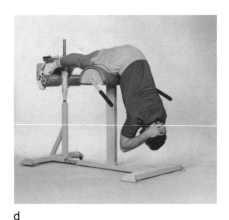

c   d

Figure 13.22   (Continued)

ABDOMINAL/OBLIQUE EXERCISES

All sports require abdominal and oblique strength for stability, bending, pulling, and twisting. Sometimes abdominal strength is confused with hip-flexor strength because the hip flexors are tied in very close in that area. Abdominal strength is usually inferior to hip-flexor strength; therefore for muscular balance the abdominals need to be strengthened independently. To strengthen this area the athlete must perform exercises that bend the trunk forward and side to side.

Sit-Up Crunch

The athlete lies back with knees bent and feet flat on the floor close to the buttocks (Figure 13.23a). Arms are crossed behind the head. For added resistance a weight plate can be held on the chest. The athlete starts to curl at the shoulders first, then upper back, then lower back (Figure 13.23b, c). Keeping the knees up and the lower back on the floor will avoid unnecessary pressure on the lower back. The curling movement should be done without jerking or twisting. At the top the athlete pauses momentarily. Most of the muscle contraction occurs during the first 50 to 60 degrees; therefore the athlete does not need to curl all the way to the knees. The athlete then lowers the torso so the lower back touches the floor first followed by the upper back. To keep constant tension, the head and shoulders should not touch the floor after the set has begun. The athlete should not relax at the bottom but keep the abdominals tight and shoulders curled inward and repeat the movement. The athlete should inhale on the way up and exhale on the way down. The feet should not be locked under equipment because this trains the hip flexors. Some athletes may not be able to do these without hooking their feet under something. As abdominal strength increases they will be able to do the regular sit-up crunch without hooking their feet.

Oblique Twists

This exercise is not for beginner athletes because it requires good abdominal and lower-back strength. Because of the position of the torso (hanging from a bench) the lower back gets a lot of stress. The athlete uses a back raise apparatus and sits on it with feet hooked under the foot supports (Figure 13.24a). The torso will be almost parallel to the floor. The athlete puts hands together and extends the arms straight over the face, then twists the torso to the right, keeping hips flat on the pad (Figure 13.24b). The athlete returns to the straight position, then twists to the left (Figure 13.24c, d). Twisting to

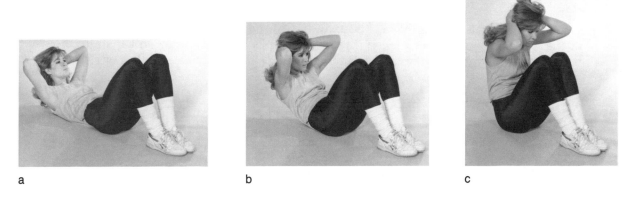

a   b   c

Figure 13.23   Sit-up crunch.

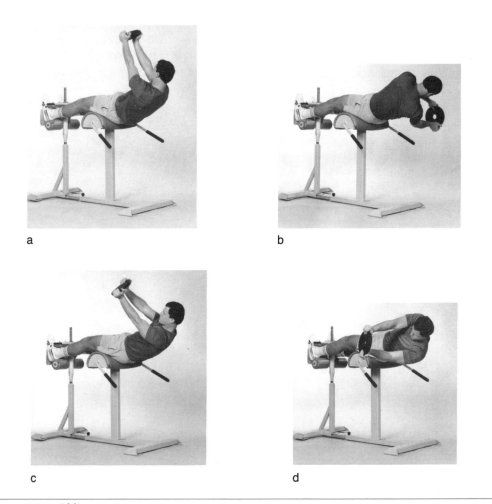

a   b

c   d

Figure 13.24   Oblique twists.

both sides and back to the starting position is one repetition. The individual's flexibility will determine how far to the side he or she can twist. For best results the athlete should keep eyes on the hands. This will cause the head to turn from side to side also. At all times the arms should extend forward. For added resistance the athlete can hold moderate weights.

LEG EXERCISES

When we refer to leg strength we almost always think of the quadricep muscle in front of the leg. The back part of the leg, the hamstring, is very important to leg strength too. Seldom referred to but almost as important is ankle and calf strength. For strong legs all those areas need to be trained.

Leg Extension

The athlete sits on the apparatus, holding on to the sides for stability (Figure 13.25a). Feet are placed under the moving pads. The knee joint should be slightly off the pad for comfort and reduced knee stress when the leg is bent. The bottom roller should be on the lower part of the shin close to the feet.

The athlete extends the legs straight forward, stops momentarily, then lowers the weight gradually to the starting position (Figure 13.25b, c). The athlete should not lower all the way but keep some tension. There should be no bouncing or jerking movements. The forward movement should be quicker than the lowering movement but still controlled. The trunk should be kept straight at all times so the quads are doing the work. The hips and torso should not move or swing to help bring the weight up. The athlete should inhale while lowering the legs, exhale when raising them.

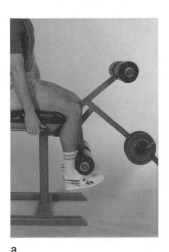
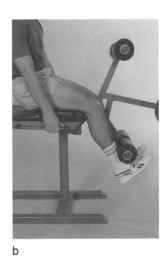
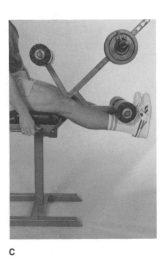

a   b   c

Figure 13.25 Leg extensions.

Leg Curl

The athlete lies face down on the machine, body straight, hands holding the side of the machine for stability. The head faces forward and knees rest off the pad so the legs can flex easily without putting pressure on the patella tendon (Figure 13.26a). The athlete's feet are under the pad with the pad resting on the Achilles tendon area. The athlete pulls the weight up by flexing at the knees so the pads almost touch the buttocks (Figure 13.26b, c). The athlete should not lift the hips because this allows the hip muscles to pull the weight up. When top position is reached, the athlete stops momen-

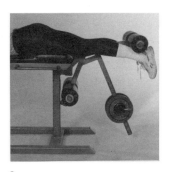
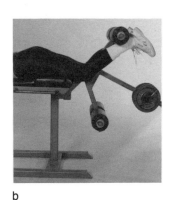
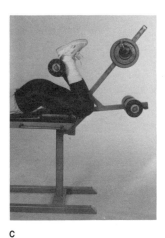

a   b   c

Figure 13.26   Leg curls.

tarily, then slowly lowers the pads to the starting position. At the bottom the legs do not relax but keep some tension. The weight should not be bounced at the bottom and the torso should remain still, with the only movement at the knees. The athlete should inhale when lowering, exhale when raising.

The leg curl strengthens the hamstrings. Many hamstring injuries occur because athletes have not put much emphasis on strengthening this muscle and too much emphasis on the quadriceps, the powerful extensor muscles of the legs. A general basic strength ratio between the two muscle groups is 2:1. In other words, the athlete should be able to do two times as much weight in the leg extension as in the leg curl.

Standing Heel Raises

Standing heel raises work the calf muscles, which extend from the ankle to the knee. Also trained are the Achilles tendons, helping them to be more flexible and to move in a full range of motion. This exercise also works all the muscles and tendons around the ankle, giving strength and flexibility in that area.

The bar should rest high on the shoulders. Hands hold on to the bar with the elbows pointing down, head looking up, and body straight (Figure 13.27a). With the weight resting on the shoulders the athlete steps up on the wood block. All the weight is supported on the toes and balls of the feet. The feet should be 8 to 12 inches apart, pointing straight forward. In this position the athlete extends straight up as high as possible, keeping the legs straight and the knees locked (Figures 13.27b, c). The athlete stops momentarily at the top, then slowly lowers the heels lower than the block to get a good stretching effect (Figure 13.27d). The depth at the bottom position will depend on ankle flexibility. The more the exercise is done, the farther down the athlete is able to go because ankle flexibility is improved.

The exercise can also be performed with a variety of machines and with the athlete standing or sitting.

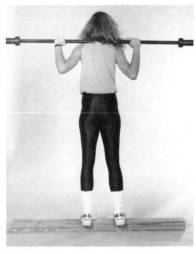

a

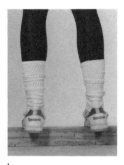

b

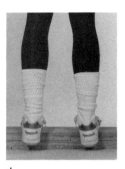

c

d

Figure 13.27 Standing heel raises.

Appendix A

Percentage Tables
(Note: Rounded to nearest 5 pounds)

Weight	40%	45%	50%	55%	60%	65%	70%	75%	80%	85%	90%	95%
100	40	45	50	55	60	65	70	75	80	85	90	95
110	45	50	55	60	65	70	75	85	90	95	100	105
120	50	55	60	65	70	80	85	90	95	100	110	115
130	55	60	65	70	80	85	90	100	105	110	115	125
140	55	65	70	75	85	90	100	105	110	120	125	135
150	60	70	75	85	90	100	105	115	120	130	135	145
160	65	75	80	90	95	105	110	120	130	135	145	150
170	70	80	85	95	100	110	120	125	135	145	155	160
180	70	80	90	100	110	115	125	135	145	155	160	170
190	75	85	90	105	115	125	135	145	150	160	170	180
200	80	90	100	110	120	130	140	150	160	170	180	190
210	85	100	105	115	125	135	145	155	170	180	190	200
220	90	100	110	120	130	145	155	165	175	185	200	210
230	95	105	115	125	140	150	160	175	185	195	205	220
240	95	110	120	130	145	155	170	180	190	205	215	230
250	100	115	125	140	150	165	175	190	200	215	225	240
260	105	120	130	145	155	170	180	195	210	220	235	245
270	110	125	135	150	160	175	190	200	215	230	245	255
280	110	125	140	155	170	180	195	210	225	240	250	265
290	115	130	145	160	175	190	205	220	230	245	260	275
300	120	135	150	165	180	195	210	225	240	255	270	285
310	125	140	155	170	185	200	215	230	250	265	280	295
320	130	145	160	175	190	210	225	240	255	270	290	305
330	135	150	165	180	200	215	230	250	265	280	300	315
340	135	155	170	190	205	220	240	255	270	290	305	325
350	140	160	175	195	210	230	245	265	280	300	315	335
360	145	160	180	200	220	230	250	270	290	310	320	340

(Cont.)

Percentage Tables (Continued)

Weight	40%	45%	50%	55%	60%	65%	70%	75%	80%	85%	90%	95%
370	150	170	185	205	220	240	260	280	295	315	330	350
380	150	170	190	210	230	250	265	285	305	325	340	360
390	160	180	200	210	230	250	270	290	310	330	350	370
400	160	180	200	220	240	260	280	300	320	340	360	380
410	165	185	205	225	245	265	285	310	330	350	370	390
420	170	190	210	230	250	270	290	320	340	360	380	400
430	170	195	215	235	260	280	300	320	345	365	390	410
440	175	200	220	240	265	285	310	330	350	375	395	420
450	180	200	230	250	270	290	320	340	360	380	410	430
460	185	210	230	250	275	300	320	345	370	390	415	440
470	190	210	235	260	280	305	330	350	375	400	425	445
480	190	220	240	260	290	310	340	360	380	410	430	460
490	195	220	245	270	295	320	345	370	395	415	440	465
500	200	225	250	275	300	325	350	375	400	425	450	475
510	200	230	260	280	310	330	360	380	410	430	460	490
520	210	235	260	285	315	340	365	390	415	440	470	495
530	210	240	265	290	320	345	370	400	425	450	480	505
540	220	240	270	300	320	350	380	410	430	460	490	510
550	220	250	275	300	330	360	385	410	440	465	495	520
560	225	250	280	310	335	365	390	420	450	475	505	530
570	230	260	290	310	340	370	400	430	460	480	510	540
580	230	260	290	320	350	375	405	435	465	490	520	550
590	235	265	295	325	355	385	415	440	470	500	530	560
600	240	270	300	330	360	390	420	450	480	510	540	570

Appendix B

Core Exercise Weight Progression Chart

Set 1	Set 2	Set 3	Set 4	Set 5	Set 6
75	85	95	105	115	125
75	85	95	110	120	130
75	90	105	115	125	135
75	90	105	120	130	140
85	95	110	125	135	145
85	95	110	130	140	150
85	105	115	135	145	155
85	105	115	135	150	160
95	110	125	140	155	165
95	110	125	140	155	170
95	115	130	145	160	175
95	115	130	150	165	180
95	125	140	155	170	185
95	125	140	160	175	190
95	135	150	165	180	195
95	135	150	170	185	200
135	145	160	175	190	205
135	145	160	180	195	210
135	155	170	185	200	215
135	155	170	190	205	220
135	155	180	195	210	225
135	155	180	200	215	230
135	155	185	200	215	235
135	155	185	205	220	240
135	155	185	205	225	245
135	155	185	210	230	250
135	155	185	215	235	255
135	155	185	220	240	260
135	155	185	225	245	265
135	155	185	230	250	270
135	155	195	235	255	275
135	155	195	240	260	280
135	185	225	245	265	285
135	185	225	250	270	290
135	185	225	255	275	295
135	185	225	260	280	300
135	185	225	265	285	305
135	185	225	270	290	310
135	185	225	275	295	315
135	185	225	280	300	320

(Cont.)

Core Exercise Weight Progression Chart (Continued)

Set 1	Set 2	Set 3	Set 4	Set 5	Set 6
135	185	245	285	305	325
135	185	245	290	310	330
135	225	255	295	315	335
135	225	255	300	320	340
135	225	255	305	325	345
135	225	255	310	330	350
135	225	275	315	335	355
135	225	275	320	340	360
135	225	275	325	345	365
135	225	275	325	350	370
135	225	275	330	355	375
135	225	275	335	360	380
135	225	275	335	365	385
135	225	275	340	370	390
135	225	315	345	375	395
135	225	315	350	380	400
135	225	315	355	385	405
135	225	315	360	390	410
135	225	315	365	395	415
135	225	315	370	400	420
135	225	315	375	405	425
135	225	315	380	410	430
135	225	315	380	415	435
135	225	315	385	415	440
135	225	315	385	415	445
135	225	315	390	420	450
135	225	315	390	420	455
135	225	315	395	430	460
135	225	315	400	435	465
135	225	315	405	440	470
135	225	315	405	445	475
135	225	315	415	450	480
225	315	365	425	455	485
225	315	365	430	460	490
225	315	365	435	465	495
225	315	365	440	470	500
225	315	365	445	475	505
225	315	365	450	480	510
225	315	405	455	485	515
225	315	405	460	490	520
225	315	405	465	495	525
225	315	405	465	500	530
225	315	405	465	505	535
225	315	405	470	510	540
225	315	405	475	515	545
225	315	405	480	520	550
225	315	405	485	525	555
225	315	405	485	525	560
225	315	405	485	525	565
225	315	405	490	530	570
225	315	405	495	540	580
225	315	405	495	545	585
225	315	405	495	550	590
225	315	405	500	555	595
225	315	405	500	560	600

Appendix C

Auxiliary Exercise Weight Progression Chart

Set 1	Set 2	Set 3
5	5	5
5	10	10
5	10	15
10	15	20
15	20	25
20	25	30
25	30	35
30	35	40
30	40	45
35	45	50
40	50	55
40	50	60
45	55	65
50	60	70
55	65	75
60	70	80
65	75	85
70	80	90
75	85	95
80	90	100
85	95	105
85	95	110
85	100	115
90	105	120
95	110	125
100	115	130
105	120	135
110	125	140

(Cont.)

**Auxiliary Exercise Weight Progression
Chart** (Continued)

Set 1	Set 2	Set 3
110	130	145
110	135	150
115	135	155
120	140	160
125	145	165
130	150	170
135	155	175
135	160	185
145	170	190
145	175	195
145	175	200
145	175	205
155	185	210
155	185	215
155	190	220
155	195	225
165	200	230
165	205	235
175	210	240
175	215	245
185	220	250
185	225	255
185	230	260
195	235	265
195	240	270
205	245	275
205	245	280
205	245	285
205	255	290
205	255	295
215	265	300
215	265	305
225	275	310
225	275	315

Additional Resources

Bliss, S. (1986). *Buckeye football fitness*. Champaign, IL: Leisure Press.

Fleck, S.J., & Kraemer, W.J. (1987). *Designing resistance training programs*. Champaign, IL: Human Kinetics.

Harre, D. (1982). *Principles of sport training*. Berlin: Sport Verlag.

Lander, J.E. (1986). Why use a belt? *Strength-Power Update*, **1**.

Martens, R. (1987). *Coaches guide to sport psychology*. Champaign, IL: Human Kinetics.

National Strength and Conditioning Journal. Published bimonthly by the National Strength and Conditioning Association, Lincoln, Nebraska.

Orlick, T. (1980). *In pursuit of excellence*. Champaign, IL: Human Kinetics.

Scholick, M. (1986). *Circuit training*. Berlin: Sport Verlag.

Sharkey, B.J. (1990). *Physiology of fitness* (3rd ed.). Champaign, IL: Human Kinetics.

Sorani, R. (1966). *Circuit training*. Dubuque, IA: Brown.

Strength Tech, Inc. (1989, May). *Institutional weight room design manual*. Author.

Glossary

active rest—The strength training period in which the athlete reduces the amount of strength training performed or does other physical activities to maintain strength and allow the body to recuperate.

antagonistic muscles—The muscles on the side of the joint opposite from the muscles being worked.

apparatus—In this text refers to exercise machines or equipment.

auxiliary exercise—Exercise that works a specific muscle or groups of muscles to complete total-body strength or to isolate a specific muscle area.

biomechanical specificity—Strength training exercises that duplicate movement used during the sport activity.

C.S.C.S.—Certified Strength and Conditioning Specialist.

circuit strength training—A training program in which the exercise stations are arranged so the athlete can move quickly from one to another and work alternate muscle groups.

collar—A clamp that secures plates to the bar.

concentric contraction—The contraction of muscle as it exerts force against a resistance.

contraction—The reaction of the muscle as it works against a resistance. A shortening of the length of a muscle.

cool-down—Easy exercises to bring the body back to pre-training status.

core exercises—Exercises that work the main muscle groups and serve as a base for all strength training programs.

double pyramid—Extra sets using progressively less weight; performed after reaching the heaviest weights.

eccentric contraction—The contraction of muscle as it resists a force.

endurance—The ability of muscle to withstand continued stress.

endurance sports—Those sports requiring athletes to exert energy continuously with little rest intervals.

estimated personal best—Using the weight performed for several reps along with a formula to get the approximate equivalent of one repetition max (1RM).

explosive movement—Movement done vigorously for a very short duration.

extrinsic motivation—Motivation coming from factors outside the athlete.

failure, training to—Doing a certain number of repetitions until the body can temporarily do no more.

flexibility—The athletic ability to extend, move, or rotate body parts in full range of motion.

free weights—Barbells and dumbbells that can be used many ways without restrictions.

frequency—The number of times per week, day, or season the athlete trains.

full range of motion—The greatest range of movement a muscle or body part can achieve.

hyperextension—The extension of a muscle beyond its normal extension.

hypertrophy—The increased size of muscle gained through exercise or strength training.

in-season training—Strength training performed during the competition season to maintain strength levels.

intensity—How heavily an exercise is performed.

intrinsic motivation—Motivation coming from within the athlete.

isolate—The ability to zero in on a specific muscle.

joint stability—The strength of a body joint due to strength training.

lift-off—Help given by a spotter (partner) to unrack the bar.

load—The amount of weight (resistance) the athlete is using during exercise execution.

lower-body exercises—Strength training exercises that work the main muscle groups of the lower body.

manual resistance—Exercises done while a partner applies resistance.

max—The most an athlete can lift in a particular exercise.

metabolic specificity—Specificity of training based on the energy system being trained.

motivation—Any stimulus (extrinsic or intrinsic) that encourages the athlete to continue toward a set goal.

multijoint exercises—Those exercises that work several body parts and large muscle groups simultaneously.

muscle fatigue—Condition of the body after strenuous training.

muscular balance—The maintenance of the natural strength ratio between opposing muscle groups.

muscular endurance—The muscles' ability to withstand isolated or overall effects of fatigue on the body during prolonged work or competition. See Endurance.

N.S.C.A.—National Strength and Conditioning Association.

negative training—Using heavier weight on the down part of an exercise.

off-season training—The period the athlete is not in sport competition but is strength training to bring strength to a higher level.

overload principle—A system of giving the body loads greater than it is accustomed to in order to increase strength.

overtraining—A point in strength training where the athlete reaches a plateau or reduction in performance.

power—The ability of a muscle to contract forcefully and exert maximum force.

preseason—The strength training period just before the sport season begins and in which the athlete should be at his or her optimal strength level.

prescribed workout—The workout assigned to the athlete, including the exercises, weights, sets, and reps.

progressive resistance—A strength training system that progressively and gradually increases the resistance (weight) the athlete uses toward greater strength gains.

pyramid system—A strength training program in which the athlete performs a number of sets with increasing weight loads and decreasing repetitions.

recovery—The time necessary for muscles to recuperate after a workout.

repetitions—The number of times an exercise movement is repeated.

repetitions maximum (RM)—The maximum weight that can be used for a specific number of repetitions.

resistance—The weight the athlete is moving to perform the exercise.

rest—The duration of time given between sets or workouts to allow for muscle recovery.

set—A group of repetitions of the same exercise and weight.

split routine—A program that works half the body parts on one day and the other half on another day.

spotters—Assistants who stand by to assist the trainee in the event of an unsuccessful attempt, to offer encouragement, and to maintain safety.

spotting techniques—Variations of spotting depending on the exercise performed.

sticking point—The point at which the body biomechanically has least advantage in moving the weight.

strength level—How strong an athlete is, based on the length of time the athlete has been training.

strength training technique—The proper method of performing an exercise to improve strength and avoid injury.

submaximum load—A resistance less than the maximum a muscle can withstand.

testing—The period in which an athlete's strength progress is evaluated.

total-body exercises—Exercises that train many muscles in the lower and upper body simultaneously.

total-body routines—A strength training routine that trains the whole body on each workout day.

utility bench—A flat bench used in various exercises.

variable resistance machines—Machines that consist of cams or leverages and that can change the actual resistance throughout the full range of motion.

volume—The total work performed during training per workout, week, or season.

warm-up sets—The performance of exercise with lighter weight before exercising with heavier weights.

weight progression—Systematic way of increasing the weight from one set to the next.

weight room flow—The circulation of athletes from one apparatus or station to another during a workout.

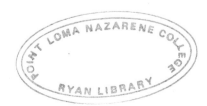